Pharmaceutical Marketing

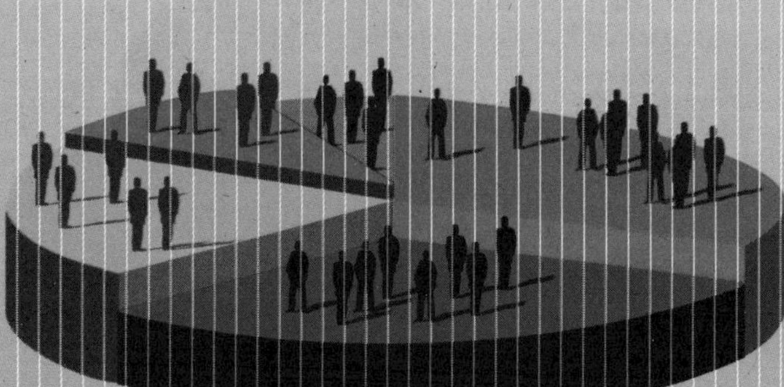

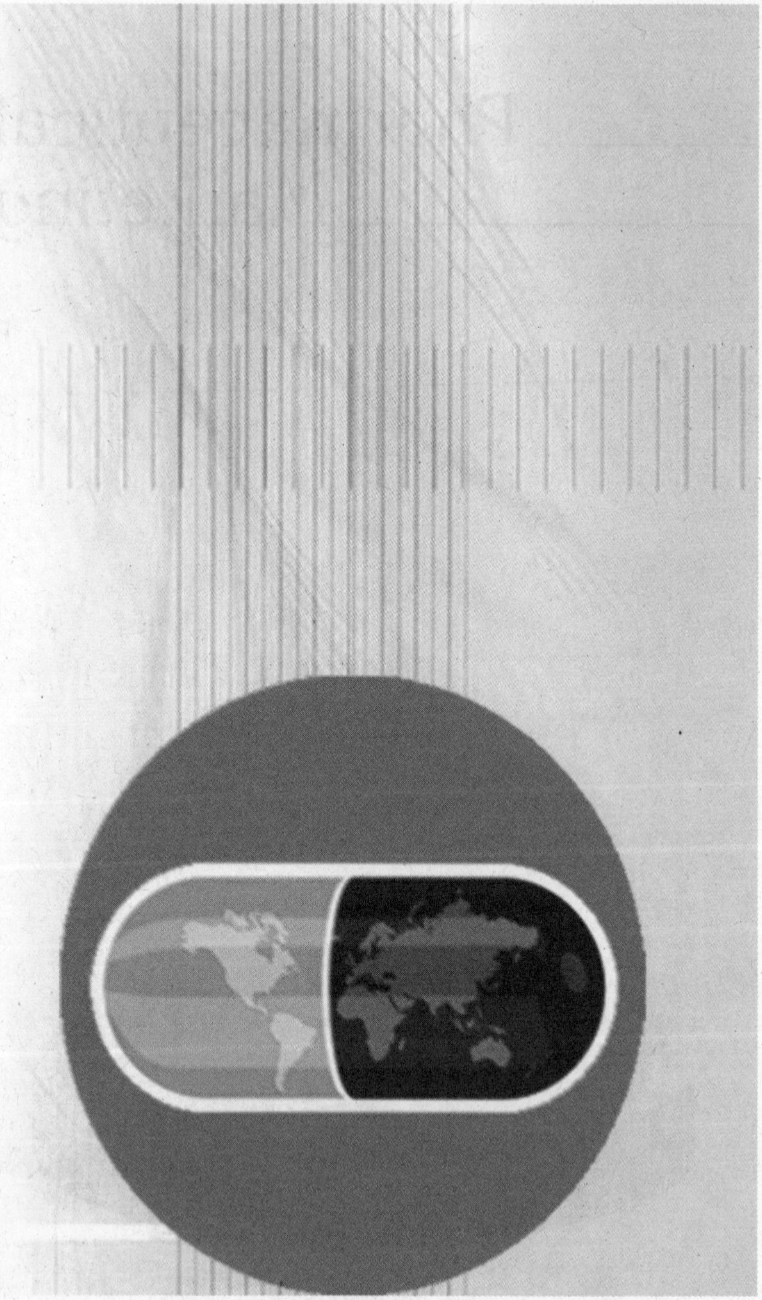

Pharmaceutical Marketing

Ajoy S. Joseph MBA PhD

Professor and Head
Department of Management Studies
Srinivas Institute of Technology
Mangalore, Karnataka

CBS Publishers and Distributors Pvt Ltd
New Delhi • Bengaluru • Pune • Kochi • Chennai

Disclaimer

Science and technology are constantly changing fields. New research and experience broaden the scope of information and knowledge. The author has tried his best in giving information available to him while preparing the material for this book. Although, all efforts have been made to ensure optimum accuracy of the material, yet it is quite possible some errors might have been left uncorrected. The publisher, printer and the author will not be held responsible for any inadvertent errors or inaccuracies.

Pharmaceutical Marketing

ISBN: 978-81-239-1902-7

First Edition: 2010

Published by Satish Kumar Jain and produced by Vinod K. Jain for
CBS Publishers & Distributors Pvt Ltd
4819/XI Prahlad Street, 24 Ansari Road, Daryaganj,
New Delhi 110 002, India.
Ph: 23289259, 23266861/67 Fax: +91-011-23243014
Website: www.cbspd.com
e-mail: delhi@cbspd.com; cbspubs@vsnl.com; cbspubs@airtelmail.in.

Branches

- Bengaluru: Seema House 2975, 17th Cross, K.R. Road, Banasankari 2nd Stage, Bengaluru 560 070, Karnataka
  Ph: +91-80-26771678/79 Fax: +91-80-26771680 e-mail: bangalore@cbspd.com
- Pune: Bhuruk Prestige, Sr. No. 52/12/2+1+3/2 Narhe, Haveli (Near Katraj-Dehu Road Bypass), Pune 411 051, Maharashtra
  Ph: -20-32404169 e-mail: pune@cbspd.com
- Kochi: 36/14 Kalluvilakam, Lissie Hospital Road, Kochi 682 018, Kerala
  Ph: +91-484-4059061-65 Fax: +91-484-4059065 e-mail: cochin@cbspd.com
- Chennai: 20, West Park Road, Shenoy Nagar, Chennai 600 030, Tamil Nadu
  Ph: +91-44-26260666, 26208620 Fax: +91-44-45530020 email: chennai@cbspd.com

Printed at Paras Offset Pvt Ltd, C-176, Naraina Industrial Area Phase-I, New Delhi

to

my beloved father
Late Prof C.T. Joseph

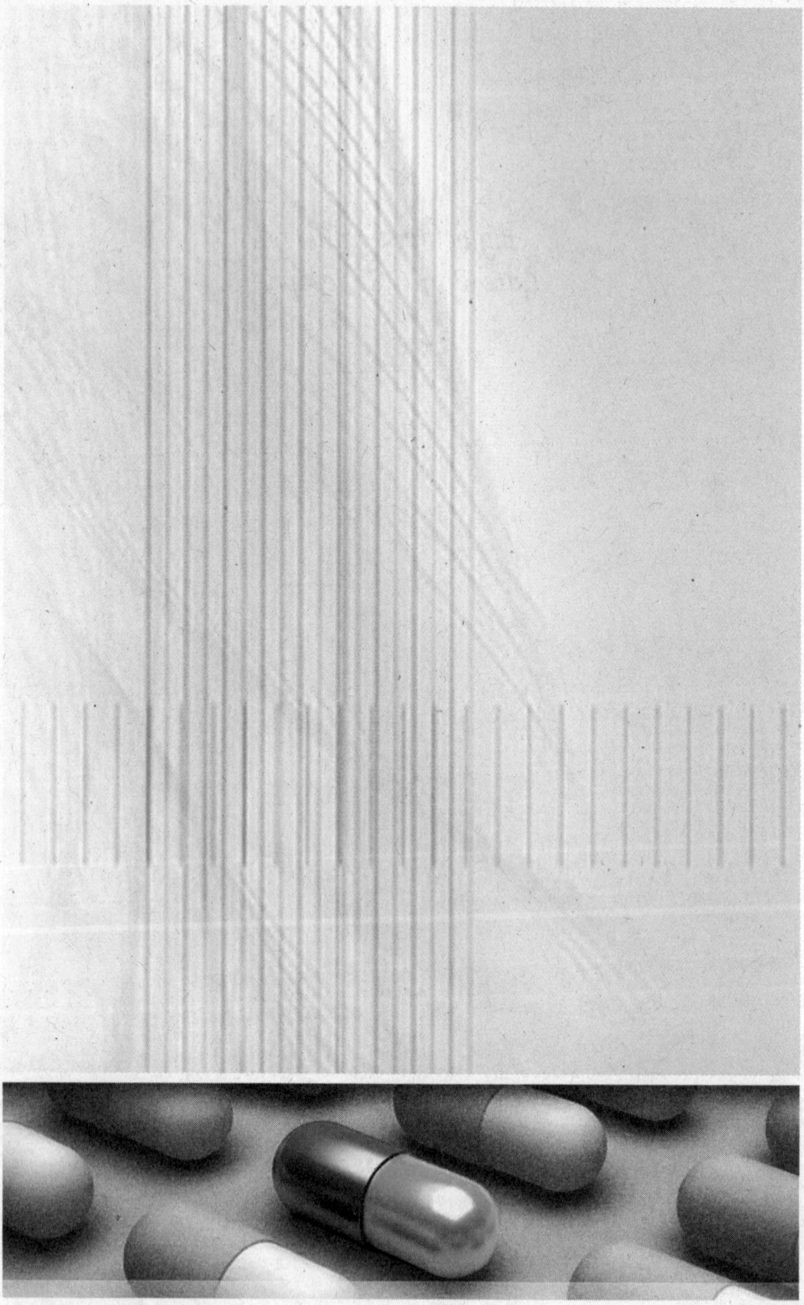

Preface

Pharmaceutical Marketing will serve as a textbook on marketing of pharmaceutical products for graduate and postgraduate students pursuing courses in marketing management in general and pharmaceutical marketing in particular. This book is beneficial to pharmaceutical marketers, medical representatives and research scholars.

The book provides an overview of Indian pharmaceutical industry, global pharmaceutical industry and the US pharmaceutical industry. It covers basic marketing concepts, marketing planning process, and prescribing behaviour. The book also covers in detail about each of the marketing mix elements of pharmaceutical marketing.

Ajoy S. Joseph

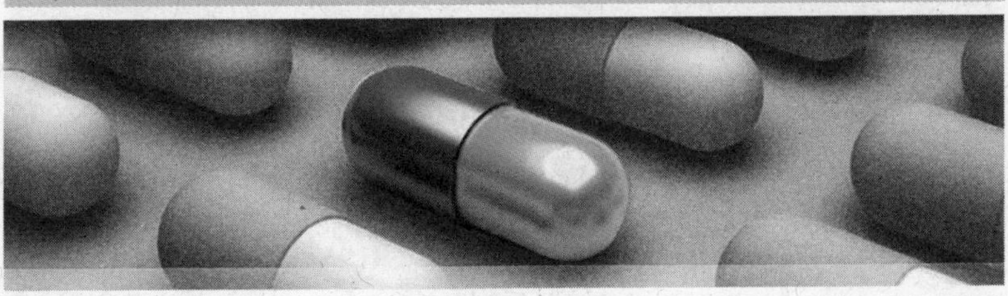

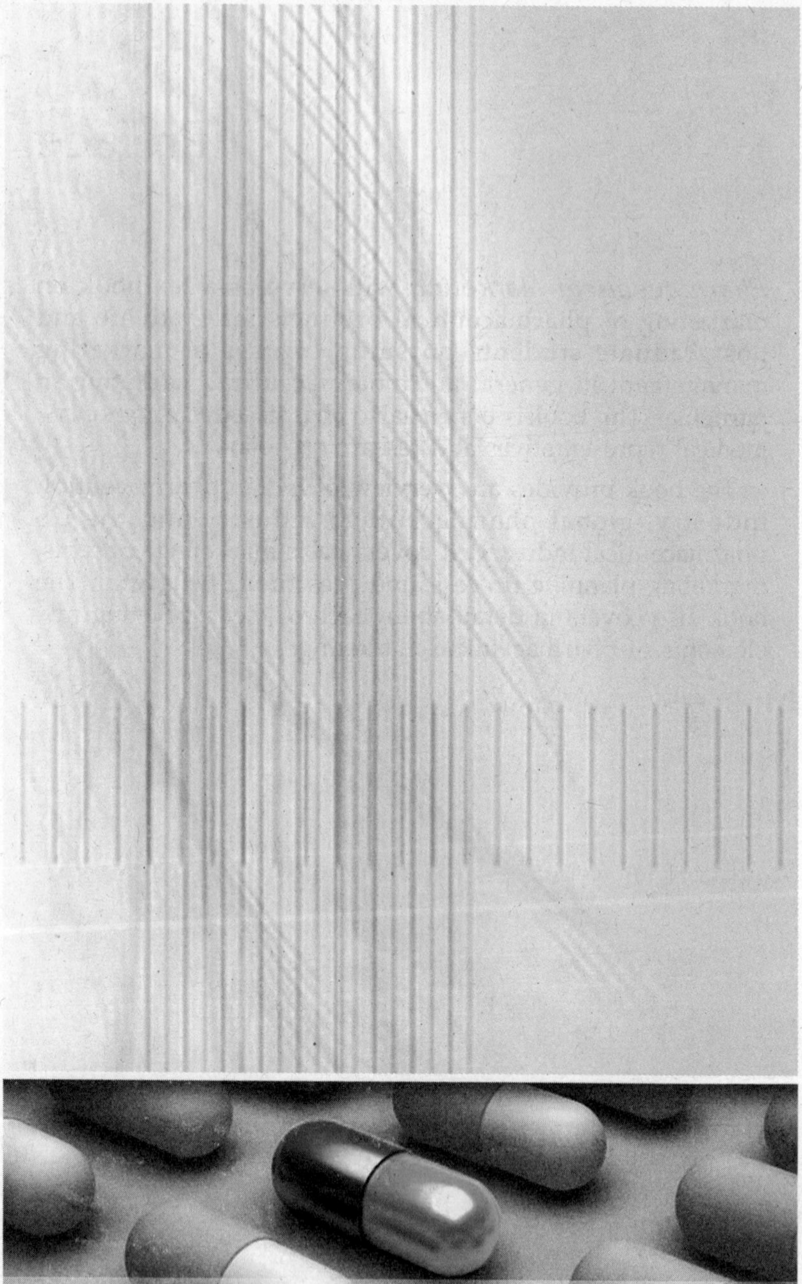

Contents

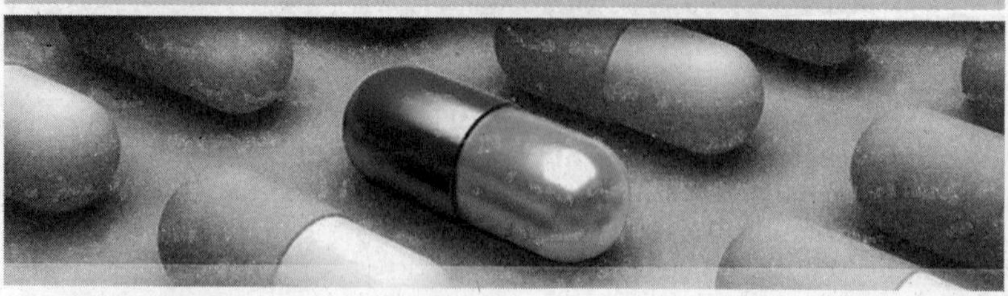

1 Indian Pharmaceutical Industry: An Overview

The pharmaceutical industry develops, produces, and markets medicinal drugs. Pharmaceutical companies can deal in generic and/or brand medications. They are subject to a variety of laws and regulations regarding the patenting, testing and marketing of drugs.

Indian Pharmaceutical industry has more than 23,000 companies comprising of large, big, medium and small companies. India has one of the fastest growing pharmaceutical markets in the world. The Indian pharmaceutical industry, now a $17 billion (over Rs. 68,000 crore) Industry, has shown tremendous progress in terms of infrastructure development, technology base creation and a wide range of products. The Indian pharma market is currently estimated at 8.7 bn and is expected to reach 10 bn by the end of 2009, with the sectors contributing to GDP being 1.3%. Research and Development spending by the Indian pharma companies is 2–4% of sales. This is marginal compared to 10–15% of sales for the global players. Pharma companies have posted 23% growth in their revenues and 38% growth in profits. The country ranks 17th in terms of export value of bulk actives and dosage forms. Indian exports are destined to more than 200 countries around the globe including highly regulated markets of US, Europe, Japan and Australia.

The pharmaceutical industry produces bulk drugs belonging to major therapy groups. Globally the Indian pharmaceutical industry ranks 4th in terms of volume (with an 8% share in global sales), 13th in terms of value (with a share of 1.5% in global sales) and produces 20–24% of the world's generic drugs (in terms of value). The industry has developed Good Manufacturing Practices (GMP) facilities for the production of various dosage forms.

India is emerging as the global hub for contract research and manufacturing services due to a combination of low-cost and world-class quality standards. According to a study by Ernst & Young, the total market for clinical research activities in India is expected to touch $1.5–2 billion by 2010. Also, AT Kearney has listed India second (just after China) for attractiveness as a clinical trials centre. With pharma majors facing increased pressure on profit margins, spiralling R&D costs and increasing overheads, outsourcing of clinical research processes to third parties in developing countries seems a viable option. By contracting such work to India, they save 40–60% in new drug development.

India has the capability to become a global pharma hub by exporting domestically produced generic products and positioning itself as an off shoring destination for clinical and preclinical research and other support services. There is tremendous potential in the Indian pharma market itself. Consumer spending on healthcare went up from 4% of GDP in 1995 to 7% in 2007. That number is expected to rise to 13% of GDP by 2015.

In the recent past much of the profits were mostly generated by overseas operations rather than domestic sales. As the domestic pharma sector is highly fragmented most of the Indian companies are emphasizing on exports. Due to depreciation of the rupee, pharma companies have been benefited largely as they are earning most of their revenues from export sales. The progressive trend in this sector is expected to continue, due to increased integration with global trade, which began with the signing of the General Agreement on Tariffs and Trade (GATT) in January 2005. India started to recognize global patents and the growing significance of the country in terms of contract research and clinical trials.

Driven by a huge patient base, increasing incomes, improving healthcare infrastructure and strong penetration of health insurance, the pharmaceutical market is expected to grow more than double its size in the next five years. Drugs for acute diseases presently dominate this market; however, the increasing penetration of lifestyle-related diseases is expected to fuel the growth of drugs targeting chronic diseases. Growing share of the lifestyle segment in the overall pharma market has led drug companies to restructure their product portfolio to tap the huge opportunity. Companies such as Alembic in which acute therapy (anti-infectives, antibiotics) holds a dominant share have been forced to restructure their business model to focus on the lifestyle segment (cardiovascular, cancer, diabetes). To consolidate its presence in this segment, the company acquired the non-oncology portfolio, which includes cardiovascular, diabetes and gastrointestinal therapies from Dabur Pharma in 2007. The acquired businesses had gross sales of over Rs. 95 crore during 2007-2008. The lifestyle segment (chronic diseases) is growing double digit and faster than all other areas in the pharma market.

The Indian pharmaceutical market at present is highly fragmented, with the top three companies having a market share of around 5 to 7% each. However, introduction of the product patent regime is likely to result in heavy consolidation in future.

The product patent regime encourages Indian companies to invest more in Research and Development. The Indian Pharmaceutical Industry today is in the front rank of India's science-based industries with wide ranging capabilities in the complex field of drug manufacture and technology. A highly organized sector, the Indian Pharma Industry is estimated to be worth $ 8.7 billion, growing at about 8 to 9% annually and the total market is more than 37000 crores. It ranks very high in the third world, in terms of technology, quality and range of medicines manufactured. From simple headache pills to sophisticated antibiotics and complex cardiac compounds, almost every type of medicine is now made indigenously. The pharmaceutical industry in India meets around 70% of the country's demand for bulk drugs, drug intermediates, pharmaceutical formulations, chemicals, tablets, capsules, orals and injectibles. There are about 250 large units and about 8000 Small Scale Units, which form the core of the pharmaceutical industry in India (including 5 Central Public Sector Units). These units produce the complete range of pharmaceutical formulations, i.e. medicines ready for consumption by patients and about 350 bulk drugs, i.e. chemicals having therapeutic value and used for production of pharmaceutical formulations.

Following the de-licensing of the pharmaceutical industry, industrial licensing for most of the drugs and pharmaceutical products has been done away with. Manufacturers are free to produce any drug duly approved by the Drug Control Authority. Technologically strong and totally self-reliant, the pharmaceutical industry in India has low costs of production, low R&D costs, innovative scientific manpower, strength of national laboratories and an increasing balance of trade. The pharmaceutical industry, with its rich scientific talents and research capabilities, supported by Intellectual Property Protection regime is well set to take on the international market.

The Indian pharmaceutical industry is also getting increasingly US FDA compliant to harness the growth opportunities in areas of contract manufacturing and research. Indian companies such as Ranbaxy, Sun Pharma, and Dr Reddy's are increasingly focusing on tapping the US generic market. Recently, Ranbaxy Laboratories Ltd. has received a tentative approval from the US Food and Drug Administration to manufacture and market Lamivudine tablets (150 mg), a medicine used in treating HIV infection. This tentative approval has been granted under the US President's Emergency Plan for AIDS Relief Initiative (PEPFAR). In financial year 2008, imports were Rs. 20 bn while exports were Rs. 87 bn.

More than 85% of the formulations produced in the country are sold in the domestic market. Over 60% of India's bulk drug production is exported and Import of bulk drugs have slowed down in the recent years.

Pharma exports touched a level of over Rs. 24,942 crore during 2006-2007. Exports constitute a substantial part of the total production of Pharmaceuticals in India. Another noteworthy feature of export is more of dosage form export to advanced markets like Europe, US, CIS Africa, etc. The trend of exports is given in Table 1.1.

Table 1.1 The trend of exports

Year	*Exports (Rs. in Crores)*	*Year*	*Exports (Rs. in Crores)*
1998-1999	6256.06	2002-2003	12826.10
1999-2000	7230.16	2003-2004	15213.24
2000-2001	8757.47	2004-2005	17857.80
2001-2002	9751.20	2005-2006	22578.98
		2006-2007	**24942.00**

(*Source:* Directorate General of Commercial Intelligence and Statistics—GCIS, Kolkata)

Pharmaceutical Industry—Strengths

- Knowledge based industry.
- Large manufacturing base for high quality drugs and formulations.

- Developing cost effective technologies for drug intermediaries and bulk actives without a compromise on quality.
- Cost advantage in terms of drug production, maintenance of high standards in terms of purity, stability and international safety, health and environment protection.
- Tremendous export potential.
- Major driver of growth in the future.
- Strong scientific and technical manpower.
- World class national laboratories in process development.
- Increasing balance of trade in the sector.
- An excellent centre for clinical trials.
- Competencies in chemistry and process development.

The following attributes constitute the basis of the technological strengths of the Indian pharmaceutical industry.

- Self-reliance displayed by the production of 70% of bulk drugs and almost the entire requirement of formulations within the country.
- Low cost of production.
- Low R&D costs.
- Innovative scientific manpower.
- Excellent and world-class national laboratories specialising in process development and development of cost effective technologies.
- Increasing balance of trade in Pharma sector.
- An efficient and cost effective source for procuring generic drugs especially the drugs going off patent in the next few years.
- An excellent centre for clinical trials in view of the diversity in population.

The Indian government had passed Patents (Amendment) Bill on Tuesday, March 22, 2005 amid many protests from the Left parties. The passing of the bill means that India has kept its commitment to the WTO to have a product patent regime in place.

The fear that the new bill would lead to an increase in the cost of life saving drugs, is taken care off by the compulsory licensing under the bill. This will enable Indian companies to manufacture medicines for a fixed tenure in case of any epidemic, thus controlling the price factor.

The government has made crucial changes to the original draft to ensure that big pharma MNCs cannot dictate medicine prices arbitrarily. The most important change in the Act is a tighter definition of what can be patented. Now only a product, including drugs, which makes a technical advance or has economic significance, can get a patent.

Some of the changes that bill proposes include giving manufacturing rights to Indian companies, which currently produce drugs patented abroad, after paying a 'reasonable' royalty for them. The bill also restricts a pharmaceutical company from renewing its patent every time it expires, citing a new use for the same drug. It gives companies more grounds and time to challenge a patent claim even before it is granted.

The government will also have the right to issue a compulsory license to an Indian company to produce a patented product if the patent holder is charging abnormally high rates or in case of a national emergency. Expenditure on R&D by the Indian pharmaceutical companies is around 1.9% of the industry is turnover. This is very low when compared to the investment on R&D by foreign research-based pharma companies. They spend 10 to 16% of the turnover on R&D. However, now that India has entered into the Patent protection area, many companies are spending relatively more on R&D.

Playing a key role in promoting and sustaining development in the vital field of medicines, Indian pharma industry boasts of quality producers and many units approved by regulatory authorities in USA and UK. International companies associated with this sector have stimulated, assisted and spearheaded this dynamic development in the past 53 years and helped to put India on the pharmaceutical map of the world.

With the introduction of new product patent regime, MNCs have renewed their interest in India. Though, almost all the big pharma companies have their presence of India, some of the companies like Bristol Myers Squibb, Boehringer Ingelheim and Eisai have only made recent forays. Similarly Indian companies are getting ready to catch up with the global generics market $65–70 bn worth drugs are coming off patent in the US and European markets in the next two years. According to a research consulting firm, Indian drug makers will have 43% share of the global generics market by 2009 as compared to 4% today. Though MNCs are trying to corner the domestic market, Indian companies still command 70% of the domestic market.

There is an ongoing battle between MNCs and Indian firms, with both trying to eat to each other's market share. Indian players are considering acquiring assets in the US and Europe in order to grow inorganically and achieve volumes. Similarly Indian MNCs are trying to widen their distribution in overhead markets. Domestic firms are expanding globally they are first acquiring marketing facilities and later expanding into manufacturing to improve their supply chains. The core chemistry and generic products manufacturing strength of India is driving the trend. Competing in the European markets can be easy for Indian companies when compared to the US in terms of price erosion, valuations and volatility. Indian companies which are acquiring the generic pharma companies in Europe are paying 2–3 times their revenues considering this market to de-risking their business model with high risk and high return US generics market. As price pressures are mounting consolidation is rapidly taking place in the US generics market. Consequently foreign companies are also looking at Indian companies to grow inorganically. One of the key drivers for generics consolidation is the vertical integration. The Mylan acquisition of Matrix Labs exhibits the beginning of this trend. The global generic players as Teva, Abrika, Sandoz Watson, Hospira and Pliva are waiting for possible acquisition targets to strengthen their position in the global generics market while marketing India as the sourcing base. One cannot rule out that there are very few such acquisition targets in the country. For instance the Teva Aurobindo deal failed to take off and now Aurobindo is on the acquisition spree to enter the US and European markets. In the highly regulated and competitive market Indian players need to be gast and keep the costs low.

At least $1 bn has been spent on the global acquisition in the past three years by Indian companies. To fund the global acquisition and expansions, several companies have raised finances through FCCB issues last year. Mergers and Acquisitions (M&A) activity is expected to intensify as consolidation plays a crucial role in the future. Though Ranbaxy has its presence in 25 locations, the number of Indian pharma companies having their presence in multiple locations has increased to 12.

Coming under the price pressure MNC are increasingly outsourcing their manufacturing activities to low cost countries such as Indian and China. Daunted by high costs, foreign companies are outsourcing 10-15% of their production to low cost courtiers. Big pharma companies such as Merck, Glaxo and Novartis are increasingly exploring new opportunities for low cost manufacturing. The average cost reductions from sourcing manufacturing and conducting clinical trials in India is about 30–40% while it ranges form 40–60% in China. Owning the highest number of USFDA manufacturing plants outside the US India is poised to become the destination for contract to his with its new patent regime, any foreign companies are showing interest in working with Indian companies besides scouting for acquisitions. The contract research manufacturing services offer stable revenues and are less risky than generics. Indian companies such as Nicholas Piramal and Shasun Chemicals have acquired manufacturing facilities in western countries to show their long-term commitment to the market. With the new pharma and multi-product SEZs being set in India, contract manufacturing can grow significantly by leveraging the fiscal incentives to keep the cost low. One has to ensure that the time to market the drug is reduced, i.e. much before its patient expires. To reduce the time and cost big pharmas are outsourcing the clinical research to India, which is worth of $118 million per year and is predicted to reach $380 million by 2010 as more US and European companies look to Indian to costs of drug development.

Though Indian pharma companies have improved their use of technology and are moving up in value chain activities, foreign investors are still contemplating investment in India and china. This can be attributed to policy shortcomings in India, though drug prices control in India is aimed at availability of drugs to people at low costs. Pharma companies have been marred by these price regulations which are in turn affecting their profitability. Multinational drugs makers have voiced their concern to the government and have stated that they would prefer greater monitoring of drug prices to ensure that prices do not spiral out of control. Though low cost producers can cope with the new regulatory environment those who cannot produce drugs at lower cost will be forced to consolidate or stop production. Even industry experts are predicating that it is easy to grab the market, share in the US and European generics market than in the domestic market where price controls are likely to continue. Hence pharma companies have very few options left with them other than exploring export opportunities. The price controls and rising Chinese imports are likely to squeeze the margin for the domestic firms thereby forcing consolidations in the industry. In addition, the new product patient regime would change the future of the industry with the introduction of innovative drugs forcing domestic players to consolidate.

With many growth opportunities opening up, the Indian pharma sector is all set for rapid expansion. As a result the sector is currently experiencing a surge in coverage services and spending in public and private sectors. Avenues such as outsourcing manufacturing and opening up of new markets have heightened prospects for the Indian pharma market, ruining it into a land of milk and honey.

The Indian pharmaceutical sector has come a long way meeting almost 95% of the countries pharmaceutical needs. The industry is very cost effective and manufacturers drugs for less than half of the US cost and conducts R&D for less than one eight of the US cost. The global output of the industry ranks 4 in terms of volume and 13th in terms of value. It has grown at a compounded annual growth rate of 13% form 2002-2007 and is estimated to grow at a rate of 16% annually over 2007-2011. The total worth of the industry is estimated at 10 bn at present. The country has emerged as a key contrast research and manufacturer services hub and is playing a vital role in manufacturing as well as in drug development. Contrast manufacturing offers multiple opportunities.

Given the increased pressure on profit margins and increasing overheads. India is becoming a favorite R&D hot spot for global pharma companies. It is expected that with 10,000 manufacturing units by the year 2050 India will be among the top 10 nations in drug manufacturing.

Many Indian pharmaceutical majors are also showing keen interest in mergers and acquisitions as a route for growth. Some leading players are exercising the foreign currency convertible bond option as their chief acquisition currency. The companies have put in place a unique co-funding model whereby they will make any investments at the beginning and only take care of the management for a percentage share in the profits, and increase their stake slowly every year. Companies such as Alkem, JB chemicals, Sun pharmaceuticals and Indoco Remedies are entering into tie-ups will mid size US pharma companies to ease their way through the market. Research capability is also a key factor in M&A's. Dishmans acquisition of Solution pharma and Nicholas Pirammals to Avecica pharma are to acquire strong research expertise and boost the expertise through consolidation.

Likewise Cadila Healthcare Ltd's (Zydus Cadila) recent acquisition of Etna Biotech, a wholly owned Italian subsidiary of the Dutch bio-pharma company, Crucell NV, offers Cadila a research platform for developing new vaccines and technologies. Crucell, which focused on biologicals, entered the vaccine space with the acquisition of Berna Biotech, a globally renowned vaccine company. Etna was the dedicated research and development wing of Berna Biotech. Etna Biotech, headquartered in Catania, Italy, focuses on research and development of vaccines. Currently, Etna Biotech has several innovative technologies and vaccines at different development stages in its pipeline. Prominent among those are programmes for developing vaccines against Hepatitis using the virosome vaccine technology platform, and another against malaria and HPV using the measles technology platform. The need for specialized technology and cutting edge research has resulted in relatively limited competition and has posed high entry barriers for players in the field of vaccines. With the global vaccine industry forecast to grow by nearly 18% by 2010, which is roughly three times the growth of the global pharmaceutical industry, research and development of vaccines has emerged as a major focus area in recent times, and this move will help Cadila to be in the forefront of innovation for vaccine research and development.

There were M&A deals with 2.5 billion in the pharma sector in 2006 compared with just 364 million the previous year. Also on the back of a rise in ANDA approvals in US, the Indian generic drug makers are embarking on organic as well as inorganic strategies to gain a foothold in western regulated markets and semi-regulated markets of Russia, Africa, Asia and the Middle East. Dr Reddy's acquisition of Germany's Beta Pharma and Ranbaxy's acquisition of Romanians Terapia in early 2006 were the highest deals in the Indian Pharma sector. However, the acquisition could be risky especially when any problem in the acquired markets is risky for the companies' bottom lines. In the case of DRL the acquisition had resulted in the depletion of company's cash reserves and made the company incur a large debt. Further a change in the German new drug policy making 30% price cuts mandatory for generic drugs increased the pressure on the companies to reduce the prices of the drugs analysts opine, Price cuts on generics in Germany have ranged between 20–30% at a time when the overall European Pharma market itself has remained stagnant.

Investment Opportunities

- Scope for generic drug production market
- Contract research
- Lean manufacturing
- Clinical research and trials
- Significant export potential
- Supply of generic drugs to developed markets.

Research and Development

Indian pharmaceutical companies are in a favorable position to develop drugs at a fraction of the international costs due to the low manpower cost, infrastructure, quality scientists and the capability to conduct path-breaking research.

- The Government has taken various policy initiatives in order to strengthen Research and Development in the pharma sector.
- Fiscal incentives are awarded to Research and Development units in the pharma sectors towards the development of new drug molecules, clinical research, new drug delivery systems, new Research and Development set ups and infrastructure provision.
- Certain leading Research and Development companies have increased their Research and Development spending to over 5% of their turnover in comparison to an average spending of 2%.
- Pharma units interested in obtaining Income Tax Exemption under Section 35 (2AB) need to get their Research and Development unit recognized by CSIR.
- A Pharmaceutical Research and Development Promotion Fund to the tune of Rs. 150 crores has been established for promoting Research and Development in the pharma sector.

Contract Manufacturing

Many global pharmaceutical majors are looking to outsource manufacturing from Indian companies, which enjoy much lower costs (both capital and recurring) than their western counterparts. Many Indian companies have made their plants GMP compliant and India is also having the largest number of USFDA-approved plants outside USA.

Indian companies are proving to be better at developing Active Pharmaceutical Ingredients (APIs) than their competitors from target markets and that too with non-infringing processes. Indian drugs are either entering into strategic alliances with large generic companies in the world of off-patent molecules or entering into contract manufacturing agreements with innovator companies for supplying complex under-patent molecules.

Some of the companies like Dishman Pharma, Divis Labs and Matrix Labs have been undertaking contract jobs for MNC's in the US and Europe. Even Shasun Chemicals, Strides Arcolabs, Jubilant Organosys, Orchid Pharmaceuticals and many other large Indian companies started undertaking contract manufacturing of APIs as part of their additional revenue stream. Top MNC's like Pfizer, Merck, GSK, Sanofi, Aventis, Novartis, Teva, etc. are largely depending on Indian companies for many of their APIs and intermediates. The Boston Consulting Group estimated that the contract manufacturing market for global companies in India would touch $900 million by 2010.

Select Contract Manufacturing Deals in India (Table 1.2)

Table 1.2 Select contract manufacturing deals in India

Indian company	*Multinational*	*Product*
Lupin Laboratories	Fujisawa	Cefixime
	Apotex	Cefuroxime Axetil, Lisinopril (Bulk)
Nicholas Piramal	Allergan	Bulk and Formulations
	Advanced Medical Optics	Eye Products
Wockhardt	Ivax	Nizatidine (anti-ulcerant)
Dishman Pharmaceuticals	Solvay Pharmaceuticals	Eprosartan Mesylate
IPCA Labs	Merck	Bulk Drugs
	Tillomed	Atenelol

Contd...

Indian company	*Multinational*	*Product*
Orchid Chemicals and Pharmaceuticals	Apotex	Cephalosporin and other injectables
Sun Pharma	Eli Lilly	CVS products, anti-infective drugs and insulin
Kopran	Synpac Pharmaceuticals	Penicillin- G Bulk Drug
Cadila Healthcare	Altana Pharma	Intermediates for Pantoprazole
	Boehringer Ingelheim	Gastrointestinal and CVS Products
Biocon	Bristol Myers Squibb	Bulk Drugs

Export Promotion Cell

An Export Promotion cell in this sector has been incorporated with the objective of:

- Boosting Pharmaceutical exports
- Function as a nodal centre
- Promotional activities aiming at accelerating pharma exports.
- Suggestions for modifications in the EXIM Policy.
- Seminars/Workshops on standards, quality control requirements, etc.

Pharma Export Promotion Council (Pharmexcil)

The Pharma Export Promotion Council (Pharmexcil) has been constituted with the objective of:

- Facilitation of exports of Drugs, Pharmaceuticals, Biotechnology products, Herbal Medicines, Diagnostics.
- Export thrust to various products through workshops, conferences and seminars and delegate visits.

Foreign Direct Investment in Drugs and Pharmaceuticals

- Foreign Direct Investment (FDI) up to 74% in the case of bulk drugs, their intermediate Pharmaceuticals and formulations (except those produced by the use of recombinant DNA technology) would be covered under automatic route.
- FDI above 74% for manufacture of bulk drugs will be considered by the government on case to case basis for manufacture of bulk

drugs from basic stages and their intermediates and bulk drugs produced by the use of recombinant DNA technology as well as the specific cell/tissue targeted formulations provided it involves manufacturing from basic stage.

Provisions of Union Budget 2007-08 for the Pharma Sector

- Weighted deduction on in-house R&D expenditure extended for a period of five more years until March 31, 2012.
- Service Tax Exemption to DCGI2 approved CRO3s offering clinical trials for technical testing and analysis services for testing of new drugs.
- Peak customs duty reduced to 10%.
- Concessional rate of 5% customs duty plus Nil CVD on specified items extended to all research institutions registered with DSIR4.
- Additional 15 imported items for R&D purposes allowed to be imported at 5% customs duty.
- Increased budgetary allocation towards AIDS control and immunization for Polio.

Pharmaceutical Trade

- In 2005, global pharmaceutical exports totalled US$271.9 billion.
- Growth in global pharmaceutical exports has been declining since 2002. At 29.0%, growth in Australian pharmaceutical exports in 2005 was almost three times higher than growth in global pharmaceutical exports (10.0%).

GLOBAL PHARMACEUTICAL SCENERIO

Table 1.3 Global pharmaceutical sales 2000-2007

	2000	*2001*	*2002*	*2003*	*2004*	*2005*	*2006*	*2007*
Total World market (current US$)	365 bn	392 bn	428 bn	499 bn	560 bn	605 bn	649 bn	712 bn
Growth Over Previous year ($Constant US$ Growth)	11.5%	11.8%	9.5%	10.3%	8.0%	7.3%	7.1%	6.4%

Source: IMS Health Market Prognosis (includes IMS Audited and Unaudited markets)

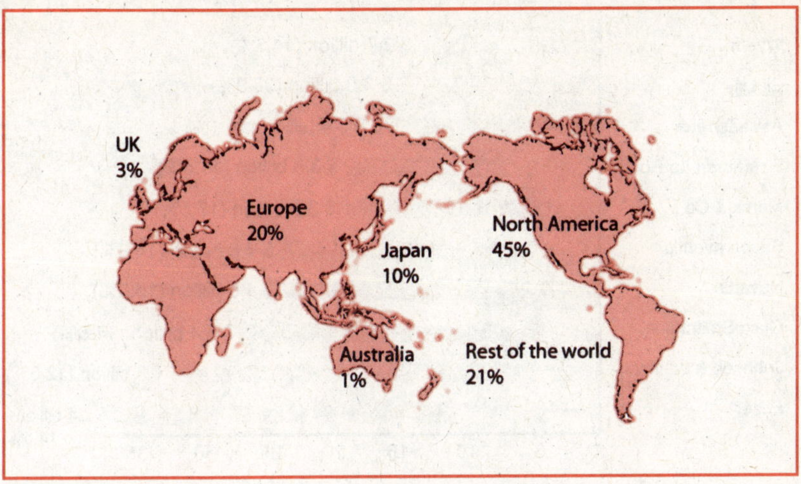

Fig. 1.1: Share of global market (sales) 2007

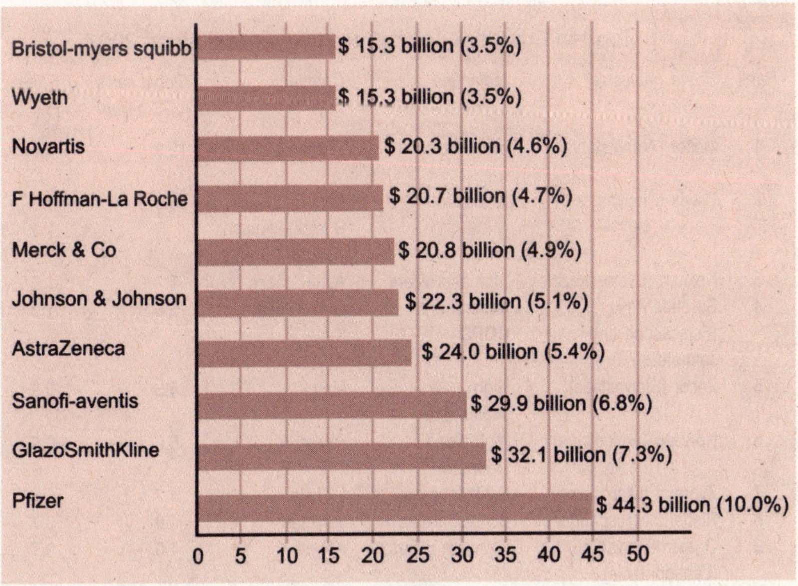

Fig. 1.2: Top ten companies worldwide by pharmaceutical sales 2007

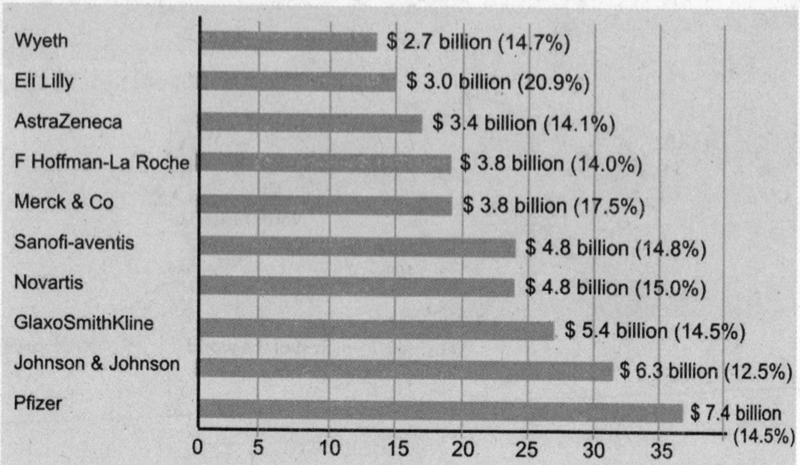

US$ billion (total R&D expenditure as % of total sales)
Source: Scrip Pharmaceutical Company League Tab les 2006 .

Fig. 1.3: Top ten pharmaceutical companies worldwide by total R and D expenditure 2007

Table 1.4 Top ten brands by global pharmaceutical sales 2007

Rank	*Brand (molecule)*	*Indication*	*Company*	*Global sales (US$ billion)*	*Share (%)*
1.	Lipitor (Atorvastatin)	High cholesterol	Pfizer	12.9	2.3
2.	Plavix (Clopidogrel)	Blood clots	Sanofi-aventis/ Bristol Myers -Squibb	5.9	1.0
3.	Nexium (Esomeprazole)	Stomach ulcers	AstraZeneca	5.7	1.0
4.	Seretide/Advair (Fluticasone and salmeterol)	Asthma and COPD	GlaxoSmith-Kline	5.6	1.0
5.	Zocor (Simvastatin)	High cholesterol	Merck	5.3	0.9
6.	Norvasc (Amlodipine)	High blood pressure	Pfizer	5.0	0.9
7.	Zyprexa (Olanzapine)	Schizophrenia	Eli Lilly	4.7	0.8
8.	Risperdal (Risperidone)	Schizophrenia	Janssen	4.0	0.7
9.	Ogastro/Prevacid (Lansoprazole)	Stomach ulcers	Abbott	4.0	0.7
10.	Effexor (Venlafaxine)	Depression	Wyeth	3.8	0.7

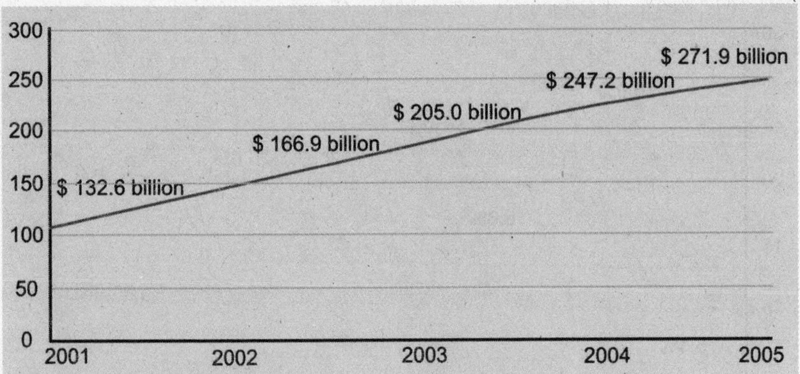

Source: World Trade Organisation, 2007.
Available: http://s tat.wto.org/StatisticalProgram /WSDBStatProgram Home.as px?Language=E.

Fig. 1.4: Global pharmaceutical exports 2001-2005

- Since 2002, annual growth of global pharmaceutical exports has exceeded growth of global exports of all manufactures; however, this margin has been decreasing over time. In 2005, growth in global pharmaceutical exports was 10.0% whilst growth in all manufactures globally was 9.9%.

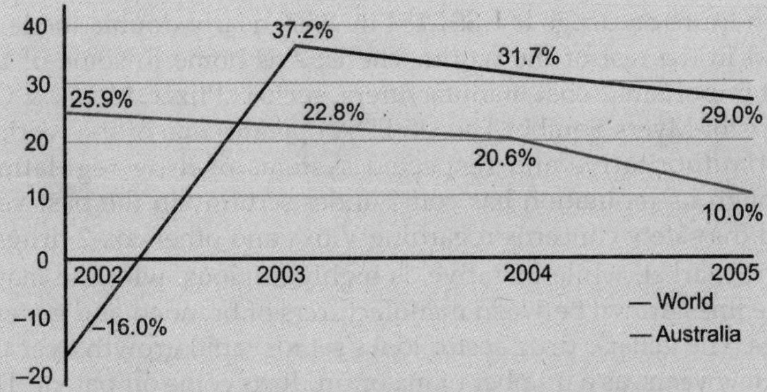

Source: World Trade Organisation, 2007. Available: http://s tat.wto.org/StatisticalProgram/ WSDBStatProgram Hom e.as px?Language=E. Please note, data in US dollars .

Fig. 1.5: Growth of global pharmaceutical exports

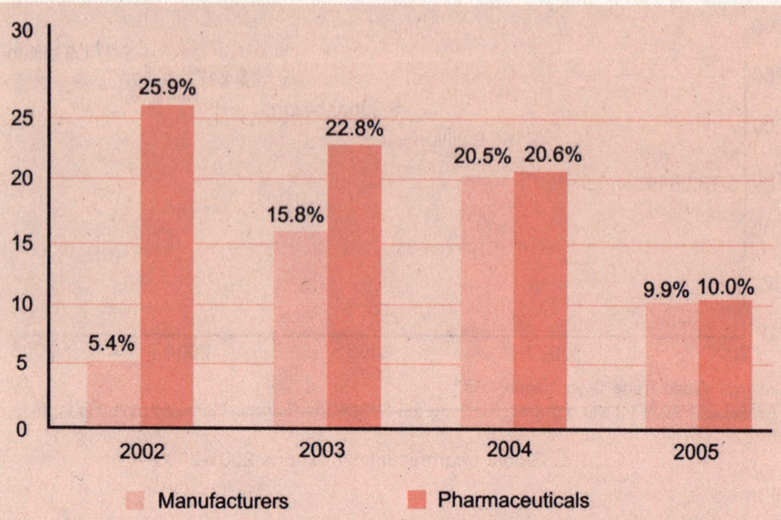

Source: WTO 2007. Available: http://s tat.wto.org/Hom e/WSDBHom e.as px?Language=E.

Fig. 1.6: Annual growth of global exports—Pharmaceuticals and manufacturing

THE US PHARMACEUTICAL INDUSTRY—A BRIEF OUTLINE

The USA is the world's largest and wealthiest pharmaceutical market, accounting for around 48% of the world total. Per capita expenditure on drugs is US$1,154 in 2007, nearly double the level found in the rest of the world. The USA is home to some of the most important global manufacturers, such as Pfizer, Merck & Co, or Bristol-Myers Squibb. The US FDA operates one of the world's most authoritative and respected systems of drug regulation, although its reputation has come under scrutiny in the past year amid the safety concerns regarding Vioxx and other cox-2 drugs.

The market, while lucrative, is highly litigious, with the major battle lines drawn between manufacturers of branded and generic drugs. The generic drug sector looks set for rapid growth over the next few years, as a number of major products come off patent. The generic industry is not without its problems, however; several companies have been under investigation for excessive price rises and collusion with branded manufacturers.

The importance of the US pharmaceutical sector is illustrated by the role it has played in the arguments over healthcare reform which have taken place since the 1990s. In November 2003, Congress finally passed legislation which will expand Medicare coverage to include prescription drugs from 2006. The Republican-inspired plan is complex and heavily weighted towards private insurance, however, and its opponents in Congress have vowed to continue to fight against it. Parallel importing of drugs was not included in the 2003 reform, but a number of state and city governments are developing plans to purchase drugs from overseas.

Table 1.5

Rank	*Theraputic class*	*Dispensed prescriptions (2006) (in million)*
1.	Anti-depressants	227
2.	Liquid regulators	203
3.	Codeine and combination	117
4.	Ace inhibitors	154
5.	Beta-blockers	130
6.	Proton pump Inhibitors	102
7.	Thyroid hormone synthetic	98
8.	Seixure disorders	95
9.	Calcium blockers	87
10.	Benzodiazepines	80
	All therapeutic classes	3707

Source: IMS Health

To provide a foundation for understanding how and why the industry in the US is changing, it is important to first consider the industry's recent past, one of the greatest periods in its history. Over the last 25 years, pharmaceutical companies have developed and brought to market a series of groundbreaking, high revenue drugs–medications that are now integral to the healthcare of million of people around the world and that have earned these organizations tens of billions of dollars. Anti-depressants, Statins, Beta-blockers, Cox-2 Inhibitors and Sexual Function Disorder treatments are just a handful of the new classes of drugs that have changed healthcare.Today more than 200 million prescriptions for statins are written each year in the US alone. Nearly 227 million prescriptions are written annually for anti-depressants. And more than 19 million Americans each year use medications to treat sexual dysfunction. This explosion in new drugs has improved the quality of life for countless people. It has likewise generated revenues for the pharmaceutical industry far greater than anyone might have imagined only a quarter century ago. Consider six of the largest pharmaceutical companies–Pfizer, Merck, Eli Lilly, Schering-Plough, Bristol-Myers Squibb, and Abbott Laboratories. In 2005 their combined revenues exceeded $137 billion and profits were about $31 billion. And in just the last 25 years, their market capitalization has grown from less than $25 billion in 1982 to nearly $525 billion by 2006.

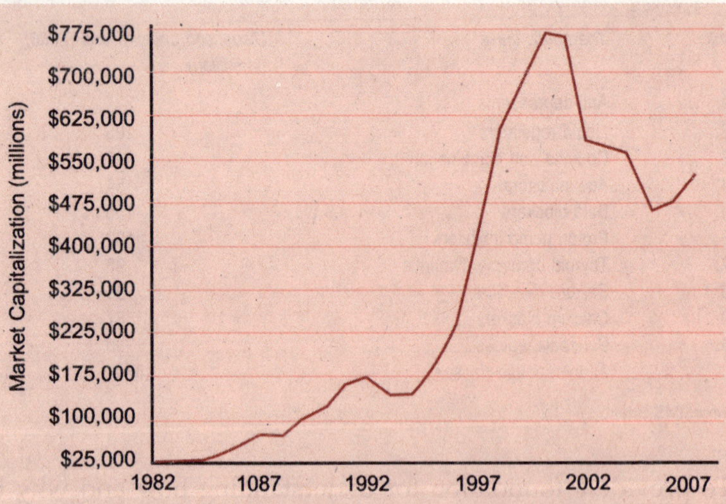

*As of 8/29/07. Aggregate capitalization of Pfizer, Merck, Eli Lilly, Schering-Plough, Bristol-Myers Squibb, and Abbott Laboratories. Source: Value Line; Yahoo Finance

Fig. 1.7: Market cap of pharmaceutical companies has grown substantially over 25 years

Forces are Changing the Industry and the Careers of its Participants

The industry, however, is on the verge of entering into a new era because a series of forces have made pharmaceutical companies' current business models obsolete. These forces can be grouped into three categories:

Revenues are Under Pressure

- ***Patents on numerous high revenue drugs are expiring:*** Major pharmaceutical companies find themselves in the unenviable position of having to rely on a small number of drugs for much of their revenue and the preponderance of their profitability. However, the patents on many of these treatments will expire over the next five years and 36 treatments that generated nearly $59 billion in US revenues in 2006 will have to compete with low-cost generic alternatives.
- ***Pipeline for new drugs looks uncertain:*** It does not appear that the drugs in the development pipelines of major pharmaceutical companies will generate anywhere near as much in revenue as those with expiring patents.
- ***More powerful payers:*** A series of mergers has created a handful of very powerful payers. Today only 10 firms control nearly 56% of the managed care market. While in the past, physicians were the key decision-makers as to which drugs were used by patients, these larger payer organizations now influence which treatments their insured will use by manipulating patient co-pays.
- ***Lower cost medications:*** Such as generics and those treatments sold by pharmaceutical companies at a below-market cost so that the payer will include them in its formulary – are provided to patients at a very low out-of-pocket cost. For all other treatments, patients must pay much more, nearly 10 times as much as the generic alternative for some drugs. Consequently, pharmaceutical companies now face the unappealing choice of having to discount even branded medications or effectively be excluded from large segments of the potential patient population.

Costs and Risks of Developing New Drugs are Increasing

At the same time that the pharmaceutical industry's revenues are under pressure, the costs and risks associated with the development of new drugs are increasing for a number of reasons.

First, many of the drugs currently under development are aimed at treating conditions that have more complex and difficult targets, thereby increasing the costs of the research process and reducing the likelihood of ultimate success.

Second, unlike in the past when the R&D process was frequently driven by obvious commercial applications, today's R&D is often driven by new scientific discoveries, a process that is far less predictable from a commercialization perspective.

Third, the regulatory approval process has become significantly more complex and costly. The regulatory agencies are more sophisticated, capable, cautious and conservative in evaluating drugs than in the past. Consequently, their standards for approvals are significantly higher. This, in turn, is forcing pharmaceutical companies to test their new treatments in larger, more comprehensive and more costly clinical trials.

Fourth, the current plaintiff-favorable litigation environment continues to be a drag on pharmaceutical company profitability. Since 2000, 65,000 product liability lawsuits have been filed against prescription drug makers–more than in any other industry. This should come as no surprise given certain features of the US tort system: plaintiffs do not need to incur any out-of-pocket costs to hire contingency-fee lawyers; prescription drug users represent a convenient group for class action certification; and unsophisticated juries are frequently willing to give exorbitant awards. Further, even if a pharmaceutical company successfully defends a lawsuit, it will incur significant legal costs in the process. Finally, payers are slowly shifting to an "outcomes-based" analysis of treatment alternatives. Under outcomes-based analysis, payers focus not on a treatment's ability to address any particular symptom, but rather its long-term effect on overall health. Consequently, predicting the potential revenue from a new treatment has become much more difficult, and it is less certain that companies who spend the hundreds of million of dollars necessary to develop new treatments will generate a sufficient return on their investments.

Globalization

The most powerful force sweeping through the industry, however, is the globalization of this industry. What had historically been a US and EU focused business is now shifting to developing countries both for the development of new treatments and as potential markets for products. The role of these countries in the development of drugs has been aided by several factors. These countries' laboratories are becoming more sophisticated as they become populated with US and EU trained scientists, and their research costs are a small fraction of their developed country counterparts. These labs also operate under regulatory regimes that encourage development through less adversarial approval processes. And the intellectual property laws of these countries are maturing.

The great economic growth experienced by developing countries has also created a much larger demand for health care and prescription medications than in the past. Although much of their near-term demand for drugs will be for generic treatments, the sheer size of the populations in these countries makes them potentially enormous markets for the industry.

Big Changes for the Pharmaceutical Industry

The confluence of these factors is compelling pharmaceutical companies to reengineer their business models, identify their core competencies and focus on what they do best. Consequently, the following trends in the pharmaceutical industry will continue, and even accelerate, in the future.

Corporate Restructuring

- ***Job reductions:*** With their revenues under pressure, pharmaceutical companies are reducing costs by shrinking the size of their workforces. From 2003 to 2006, the industry witnessed about 86,000 lay-offs. Several of the largest pharmaceutical companies have also announced plans for significant lay-offs in 2008 and 2009. This trend should continue for the foreseeable future because these companies must find ways to lower their operating costs to offset their coming drop in revenues. No one can precisely predict how many additional people will be displaced. However, two CEOs interviewed believe that "an entire generation" of *upper-middle and senior-level executives* (as many as 50,000 individuals) will be displaced.
- ***Further consolidation within the industry:*** The industry has already experienced significant consolidation. Between 1985 and the present, 51 large companies in the industry consolidated into only 10 organizations. Mergers and acquisitions between large

pharmaceutical companies will continue because they are an effective method of cutting costs. They allow the combined company to cut staffing redundancies in administrative support functions such as human resources, legal, marketing staff, senior management, and in research staff for similar product lines.

- ***Refocusing on fewer business lines:*** Another cost-cutting strategy is to spin off non-core business lines. As pharmaceutical companies narrow their focus, they are selling off entire units for treatment areas that are currently unprofitable and using the proceeds to invest in areas with greater promise and near-term potential for making money.
- ***Outsourcing:*** In addition to identifying their core business lines, pharmaceutical companies will undergo extensive reviews of their operations. They will identify those functions that allow them to most efficiently add the greatest value and try to lower their costs by outsourcing the remainder wherever possible. A key element of this strategy will be to outsource large portions of the development of new treatments to laboratories based in emerging countries. They currently operate at a fraction of the cost of those based in the US and EU, and their scientific sophistication is rapidly increasing.

Adoption of Risk Reduction Strategies

- ***Acquisitions rather than development of new compounds:*** Large pharmaceutical companies are recognizing that their strengths lie in the late stage development, commercialization and marketing of drugs rather than early stage research and development. Consequently, they increasingly are acquiring or licensing compounds developed by biotechnology companies, typically those backed by venture capital investors. Since 2001 more than $71 billion in such transactions have been completed. Today nearly 50% of the drugs marketed by large pharmaceutical companies were developed by companies or institutions other than themselves. Over time, we expect this percentage to increase significantly.
- ***Use of joint ventures and research consortiums:*** Pharmaceutical companies also are increasingly sharing the risk of developing new drugs through the use of joint ventures and research

consortiums. These partnerships involve other companies, universities, government agencies and not-for-profit entities.

Evolution of Drug Marketing

- ***Increased focus on US payers:*** As the ability of US payers to influence which drugs are used by patients increases, marketers with access to physicians will have less value than those who are sophisticated in working with payer organizations. Similarly, branding strategies and direct-consumer (DTC) marketing campaigns will focus less on a particular brand or drug than on the availability of treatments for selected conditions in general.
- ***Drugs marketed globally:*** As the demand in developing countries for prescription medications grows, pharmaceutical companies will need to recruit international sales and marketing forces. They will have to develop strategies and programs that address the unique pricing and regulatory environments of each individual country.

What Does It all Mean to an Industry Professional?

As the pharmaceutical industry adapts to the forces changing its business model, it will not only survive, but thrive. However, the adaptation process over the next five to 10 years will be very disruptive for many of its longer term employees, and will create far reaching consequences for any individual working in this field. These changes will make working at a pharmaceutical company less predictable, and individuals will increasingly need to think in terms of a career in the industry and not at just one company. And the skills in the highest demand by employers in the future will differ from those in the past. The reshaping of the industry, however, will also unlock unforeseen opportunities for those individuals who are able to anticipate the changes, prepare for and take advantage of them. Many will start new careers as independent contractors, earning far more than they ever might as an employee of a large company. Others will either start or join a new company with a unique specialty or expertise and potentially earn million of dollars should the company succeed. Still others will reposition themselves within large pharmaceutical companies to increase their importance to the enterprise and enhance their careers.

Six Future High Growth Areas of the Industry

Of the many potential opportunities, our research identified six segments of the pharmaceutical industry that we believe will offer particularly high growth potential:

Commercialization of Dormant Compounds

In the freezers of pharmaceutical companies are thousands of compounds that were abandoned prior to FDA approval, or that were approved but not commercialized. These organizations are reluctant to license or sell these compounds to other companies, largely for fear of receiving less than fair value if the drug becomes profitable for the acquiring company. Finding ways to reposition or repurpose these compounds is a high growth opportunity over the next decade because the marginal cost of doing so is a small fraction of the cost of developing a new treatment from discovery. Additionally, by repurposing a compound, a pharmaceutical company can extend the life of its patent protection.

Generic or Biosimilar Versions of Biologics

The development of generic or biosimilar versions of biologics (i.e. versions of the same treatment that are not identical to the branded medication but have enough similarity to produce comparable results in patients) will also be a high growth area. While the development and manufacture of such treatments remains difficult and expensive, the size of the market (today, 25% of the new drugs coming to market are biologics) and the near-term expiration of patents on some of the highest revenue biologics makes it a compelling opportunity. Further, recent regulatory initiatives and advances in technology have increased the likelihood that biosimilar versions of these treatments will soon be a reality.

Improving the Efficiency of R&D

The rapidly increasing costs and risks of developing drugs have led to the creation of a fast-growing business within the pharmaceutical industry finding ways to improve the efficiency of the R&D process. In particular, there will be great interest in finding ways of improving the ability to identify early in the research process (and prior to the incurrence of significant costs) those drug targets that are "inherently intractable and undruggable" or are potentially toxic to humans and therefore not viable pursuits. Additionally, because of the finite life of any drug patent, finding ways of reducing the time required from discovery through regulatory approval will be a focus of pharmaceutical companies.

Oncology and Central Nervous System (CNS) Disorders Research

As the life expectancy for the US population continues to grow, larger portions of the population will be afflicted with conditions such as Alzheimer's disease and dementia. In addition, cancer will be an even bigger cause of mortality, since for many cancers the single most important risk factor is age. As the number of those with CNS disorders and cancer increase, so too will the demand for new treatments.

Stratified Medicine and Diagnostics

While costeffective "personalized medicine" likely remains decades away, "stratified medicine"–particularly in the field of diagnostics–represents a high growth opportunity in the near-term. This field will focus on finding ways to slightly alter the composition of different medications to make them more effective for sub-segments of the patient population. The demand for new diagnostic tools in this field will grow exceptionally fast because payers view them as effective cost containment mechanisms. They also have a compelling economic model for pharmaceutical companies and venture capitalists because the regulatory approval process often can be shorter and easier than that for many drugs. Additionally, diagnostic tests are often used by much larger segments of the population than the therapeutic treatment they are designed to test for.

Fusion of Pharmaceuticals and Consumer Goods

While the regulation of consumer goods is nothing new, consumer goods companies, plagued by recent scares from poisoned dog food and toothpaste among other things, are now under far more scrutiny. They also view the areas of health and wellness products as high growth opportunities, even though such products have traditionally been the domain of pharmaceutical companies.

Consequently, consumer goods firms increasingly will seek individuals with experience in the pharmaceutical industry because of their ability to manage highly-regulated businesses and ensure product safety and efficacy.

Seven Highly-valued Skill Sets in US

These six areas will offer great growth potential and, therefore, some of the best employment opportunities over the next decade. However, the changes sweeping through the industry will also create demand from companies of all sizes for individuals with certain skills and expertise. While it would be impossible to produce an all-inclusive list of such abilities, experts believe there will be great demand for the following seven skill sets:

Ability to Manage Decentralized Intellectual Capital Resources

As more pharmaceutical companies shift to decentralized business models, they will look outside their walls for much of the intellectual capital needed to develop new drugs. Contract research organizations (CROs), independent contractors, research consortiums, universities and foreign laboratories will play increasingly integral roles in solving complex problems more cost effectively. Individuals able to simultaneously and effectively manage all of these internal and external intellectual capital resources will be in great demand across the industry.

Ability to Work in Joint Ventures and Across Divisions, Cultures and Countries

The pharmaceutical industry is shifting from fully-integrated businesses focused largely on the United States and EU markets to more decentralized business models that operate and compete in a global market. This shift will create a demand for individuals who can navigate the demands of working in joint ventures and across divisions within one company, as well as those who have the ability to work with people from different countries and cultures (which requires experience with different languages, regulatory environments and attitudes about life and work).

Ability to Integrate an Understanding of Intellectual Property Laws, Scientific Expertise and Business Strategy

Recent advances resulting from the human genome project have led to a flood of patents by companies on different gene sequences. The existence of these patents complicates the development of new drugs because it is unclear whether many (if not most) of these patents are enforceable. Consequently, there will be great demand for those individuals who can integrate an understanding of intellectual property laws (in particular, case law) with a deep understanding of science and business strategy. Such individuals will enable pharmaceutical and biotechnology companies to accurately project the potential revenue a new treatment might generate, compare it with the cost of development and thus, understand which drug development opportunities make economic sense.

Ability to Spur Creativity While Managing Commercially

In the past, pharmaceutical companies largely operated as silos – that is, each unit working on the development of a new drug largely functioned independently of the other units involved in this process. Researchers' jobs were to make scientific discoveries that would lead to new drugs. Commercialization and marketing staff were responsible for turning these discoveries into commercially viable products. The economic demands on pharmaceutical companies will force them– and all of their employees – to place a much higher emphasis on finding ways to generate revenues faster. And while these companies were able to be extremely patient in the R&D efforts in the past, hoping for a potential scientific breakthrough, they will instead be forced to more quickly terminate those projects that do not demonstrate near-term promise.

This obsession with the commercialization aspects of research and development, however, could potentially have long-term adverse effects on these organizations' ability to innovate. Scientific research is not a neat and orderly process. It requires a great deal of patience and an operating environment that encourages creativity. Absent patience and creativity, pharmaceutical company laboratories would be unable to generate the scientific breakthroughs necessary for creating new drugs. Thus, these organizations will need managers who can somehow strike a balance between two conflicting forces- instill a sense of commercial urgency in the development of new products, and do it in a way that still allows the natural creativity of the people in these laboratories to blossom.

Knowledge and Insight on the Decision-making Dynamics of Payers

The significant shift in bargaining power from pharmaceutical companies to payers has created significant demand for individuals who have a comprehensive understanding of these organizations. In particular, those people who understand not only payer business models but also how the decisions of these organizations are affected by outside influencers (employers, regulatory agencies, state and local governments, etc.) will be invaluable in determining the future pricing and positioning of drugs.

Expertise in the Functioning and Decision-making of Regulatory Agencies

One of the industry's most urgent needs is to reduce the time involved in developing and bringing new drugs to market. Regulatory agencies–both in the US and abroad—are often some of the biggest obstacles to rapidly commercialize a new treatment. Consequently, there will be great demand for regulatory specialists—that is, those individuals who have developed an expertise in how these organizations function and relationships with the individuals who work in them–who can help accelerate the approval process for a particular category of drugs.

Human Resource Skills to Help Transform Pharmaceutical Companies

Finally, as pharmaceutical companies reengineer their business models, they will need to change the types of people they recruit (and seek to retain) and the programmes in which they develop and train them. They also will need to redesign compensation structures and develop methods of encouraging behavior that is very different from how they have historically operated. Additionally, they will need to create new career paths for most significant positions in the organization. Human resources managers who can efficiently administer these changes will play a critical role in the evolution of traditional pharmaceutical companies.

Every Industry Participant will Experience Change

While there will be countless new opportunities resulting from the industry's transition, this new environment also (sadly) means that the relationship between pharmaceutical companies and their employees will change. The paternalistic environment of a quarter century ago that offered the implied promise of a safe, well-paying career at one employer as well as long-term financial well-being is economically unsustainable. Consequently, individuals who work in this industry must also recognize that they now have two businesses to run. In addition to managing their careers, they must manage their wealth. And the choices they make today will impact their financial well-being for the rest of their lives.

Career planning is also now essential to future success in this industry. As part of such a process, participants should closely study the industry so they can determine in which part they would like to work and the role they would like to play. At the same time, however, they also must recognize that the opportunities they may pursue are often constrained by financial resources and an individual's ability to bear risk. Additionally, each career choice also involves hidden costs and risks. Measuring them is an integral part of making an informed decision.

Further, just as the industry will evolve, so too will the demand for different skills and expertise. Each person should realistically assess their abilities and find ways to upgrade their value-added over time.

Successful career planning will also require personal branding strategies. Until key decision makers are aware of an individual's capabilities, that person will be afforded only limited opportunities. Thus, developing relationships with executive recruitment firms and industry peers, publishing articles and research, and participating in professional organizations are all activities that will produce great dividends for industry participants over the long term.

Additionally, the industry's coming changes will force participants to make a fundamental decision as to whether to focus their careers so that they will be viewed as 'specialists' – people with great expertise in solving particular problems – or as 'athletes'– individuals who have a broad set of capabilities and experience that allows them to manage complexity. Those who fail to do so or try to do both will soon find they are in the unenviable position of knowing too little about too much and will be of little value to most employers.

Marketing and Marketing Management

2

Marketing goes beyond a single transaction, rather the aim is to develop ties and relationships and the key to success of marketing is adopting the customers view point. Marketing is an outward looking function which tries to match the real requirements of the customer.

The starting point for the marketer is the organization itself. To get ready for the marketing orientation, the organization needs to address the following dimensions.

1. Develop an understanding of what resources the organization has at its disposal.
2. Develop a suitable filter for marketing data.
3. Use the filter to find out about the customer.
4. Review the processes to date.
5. Manipulate resources to achieve the resulting marketing objective.

By its very nature marketing has to deal with complex dimensions, particularly when addressing the following 5 main features.

1. Multiple decision makers
2. Multiple factors
3. Interaction
4. Time factor
5. Global frame

Marketing Oriented Companies

Seven common elements distinguishing marketing–oriented companies.

1. The use of market share, rather than volume, as the primary measure of marketing success.
2. The understanding and use of market segmentation principles.
3. The process for monitoring customers needs, usage, and trends as well as competitive activity – that is, market research.
4. A set of specific marketing goals and targets.
5. A structure or process for co-ordinating all non-marketing functions toward the achievements of marketing goals.
6. A corporate style and culture in which marketing integrates process participants both within and outside of the firm.
7. A market-based business concept that provides unique value to the customer.

The Marketing Mix

Product Mix

a. Product line range
b. Design concept
c. Colour appeal
d. Style
e. Package
f. Brand name
g. Service function
h. Warranties.

Distribution Mix

a. Physical distribution
b. Supplies
c. Inventory
d. Storage
e. Transportation
f. Warehousing
g. Distribution channels
h. Retailers
i. Distributors
j. Wholesalers
k. Export
l. Import.

Communication Mix

a. Advertising
b. Sales catalogue
c. Field sales force
d. Telephone sales
e. Public relations
f. Direct mail
g. Sales promotion
h. Premiums and discounts
i. Merchandising
j. Research
k. Electronic interaction.

Pricing Mix

a. Price structure
b. Payment terms
c. Costs.

Difference between Products and Benefits

Customers do not buy products, they seek to acquire benefits, lies a basic principle of successful marketing. When people purchase products, they are motivated first not by the physical attributes of the product but by the benefits that those attributes offer.

MARKETING PLAN

Marketing and Corporate Strategy

Marketing and corporate strategy are inter-related. Company's success depends on how well marketing fits into its overall corporate strategy. Marketing's input into the corporate strategy processes comprises both external and internal elements. A number of external influences affect the organization such as the prevailing social and economic climate and more directly, the accompanying legislation.

Corporate Plan

The starting point for the marketing plan and the context, within which it is set, is the corporate plan. The corporate plan is likely to contain three main components:

1. Where the organization is at present,
2. Where the organization intends to be in the future and
3. How the organization will organize its resources to get there.

Corporate Objectives

The overall objectives of commercial organizations are conventionally supposed to be financial, such as maximizing revenue, maximizing profit, maximizing return on investment or minimizing cost. However, other aims are also possible. Many companies choose long-term growth (which may be quite different form revenue maximization in the short term) Almost all have an implicit, and very powerful aim of survival which John K Galbriath spelled out so forcefully in his book the "Affluent Society". These objectives should provide a sense of purpose, help achieve consistency and provide a basis for control. To fulfill these functions, objectives should be measurable, acceptable and agreeable. It should be consistent and realistic. The objectives behind a strategy address two questions: Where do we want to be? and When do we expect to be there?

Corporate Mission

Behind the corporate objectives which offer the main context for the marketing plan, lies the corporate mission which in turn provides the context for these corporate objectives. The corporate mission can be considered as a definition of what the organization is and of what is does. This definition should not be too narrow or too wide. If it is narrow it will restrict the growth of the organization and if it is too wide it will become meaningless. Corporate mission should cover three dimensions such as customer groups or segments to be served, customer needs to be served and technologies to be utilized.

Corporate Vision

Perhaps the most important factor in successful marketing is the corporate vision. Indeed nothing drives progress like a strong vision.

Marketing Plan

A **marketing plan**, is a written document that details the necessary actions to achieve one or more marketing objectives. It can be for a product or service, a brand, or a product line. Marketing plans cover between one and five years. A marketing plan may be part of an overall business plan. Solid marketing strategy is the foundation of a well-written marketing plan. While a marketing plan contains a list of actions, a marketing plan without a sound strategic foundation is of little use.

In practice, corporate strategy and marketing are closely related, and much of the corporate strategy is derived from marketing. The development of the organization's mission and objectives largely determine its marketing strategy.

In most of the organization strategic planning is an annual process, typically covering just the year ahead. To be more effective, the plan must be formalized, usually in written form, as an identifiable marketing plan. The process typically follows a number of distinct steps. The process moves from the general to the specific, from the overall objectives of the organization down to the individual action plan for a part of one marketing programme. The marketing planning process encompasses all of the marketing skills like positioning, portfolio planning, 80/20 Rule and 4 P's .

The starting point for the marketing plan is the corporate plan. In most marketing-oriented organizations the contexts of the corporate plan will closely match those of the marketing plan itself.

How to Prepare a Marketing Plan

The main contents of a marketing plan are:

1. Executive summery
2. Situational analysis
3. Opportunities/issue analysis—SWOT analysis
4. Objectives
5. Strategy
6. Action programme (the operational marketing plan itself for the period under review)
7. Financial forecast
8. Controls.

In detail, a complete marketing plan typically includes:

1. Title page
2. Executive summary
3. Current situation—Macro environment
   - Economy
   - Legal
   - Government
   - Technology
   - Ecological
   - Sociocultural
   - Supply chain.
4. Current situation—Market analysis
   - Market definition
   - Market size
   - Market segmentation
   - Industry structure and strategic groupings
   - Porter 5 forces analysis
   - Competition and market share
   - Competitors' strengths and weaknesses
   - Market trends.
5. Current situation—Consumer analysis
   - Nature of the buying decision
   - Participants
   - Demographics
   - Psychographics
   - Buyer motivation and expectations
   - Loyalty segments.
6. Current situation—Internal
   - *Company resources*
     - Financial
     - People
     - Time
     - Skills.
   - *Objectives*
     - Mission statement and vision statement
     - Corporate objectives

- Financial objective
- Marketing objectives
- Long term objectives
- Description of the basic business philosophy.

• *Corporate culture.*

7. **Summary of situation analysis**
   • External threats
   • External opportunities
   • Internal strengths
   • Internal weaknesses
   • Critical success factors in the industry
   • Our sustainable competitive advantage.
8. **Marketing research**
   • Information requirements
   • Research methodology
   • Research results.
9. **Marketing strategy—Product**
   • Product mix
   • Product strengths and weaknesses
     - Perceptual mapping
   • Product life cycle management and new product development
   • Brand name, brand image, and brand equity
   • The augmented product
   • Product portfolio analysis
     - BCG analysis
     - Contribution margin analysis
     - Ge Multifactoral analysis
     - Quality function deployment.
10. **Marketing strategy—Segmented marketing actions and market share**
    • Objectives
    • By product
    • By customer segment
    • By geographical market
    • By distribution channel.

11. Marketing strategy—Price

- Pricing objectives
- Pricing method (e.g. Cost plus, demand based, or competitor indexing)
- Pricing strategy (e.g. Skimming or penetration)
- Discounts and allowances
- Price elasticity and customer sensitivity
- Price zoning
- Break even analysis at various prices.

12. Marketing strategy—Promotion

- Promotional goals
- Promotional mix
- Advertising reach, frequency, flights, theme, and media
- Sales force requirements, techniques, and management
- Sales promotion
- Publicity and public relations
- Electronic promotion (e.g. Web or telephone)
- Word of mouth marketing (buzz)
- Viral marketing.

13. Marketing strategy—Distribution

- Geographical coverage
- Distribution channels
- Physical distribution and logistics
- Electronic distribution.

14. Implementation

- Personnel requirements
  - Assign responsibilities
  - Give incentives
  - Training on selling methods
- Financial requirements
- Management information systems requirements
- Month-by-month agenda
  - Pert or critical path analysis
- Monitoring results and benchmarks
- Adjustment mechanism
- Contingencies (what if's)

15. Financial summary

- Assumptions
- Proforma monthly income statement
- Contribution margin analysis
- Breakeven analysis
- Monte Carlo method
- Internet strategic intelligence: ISI.

16. Scenarios

- Prediction of future scenarios
- Plan of action for each scenario .

17. Appendix

- Pictures and specifications of the new product
- Results from research already completed.

Use of Marketing Plans

A formal, written marketing plan is essential; in that it provides an unambiguous reference point for activities throughout the planning period. However, perhaps the most important benefit of these plans is the planning process itself. This typically offers a unique opportunity, a forum, for 'information-rich' and productively focused discussions between the various managers involved. The plan, together with the associated discussions, then provides an agreed context for their subsequent management activities, even for those not described in the plan itself.

Marketing Audit

As the first formal step in the marketing planning process, the marketing audit should be conducted. A marketing audit is a comprehensive systematic independent and periodic examination of a companies or business units marketing environment objectives, strategies and activities with a view of determining problem areas and opportunities and recommending a plan of action to improve the companies marketing performance.

Although some organizations employ external consultants to conduct marketing audits, they are generally best undertaken by the marketing department itself. This is mainly because they are the best open to understand the subtleties of the information revealed and moreover audit is the best possible learning process for these manages because it introduces them to the factors that are most important to the management of marketing. It also ensures that the managers who have to implement the results of the planning process understand and are committed to the assumptions that lie behind it.

Auditing Materials Includes

1. Financial data from management accounting, costing and finance departments.
2. Product data from production, R&D department.
3. Sales and distribution data from sales, packaging and distribution departments.
4. Advertising, sales promotion and merchandising data information from these departments.
5. Market data from market research department.

Analysis of Audit Material

SWOT Analysis: SWOT (Strengths, Weaknesses, Opportunities and Threats) analysis is one of the commonly used technique in the analysis of audit material. In this Internal and external factors are categorized.

Internal factors are strengths and weakness internal to the organization and its strategies and its position in relation to the competitors.

External factors are opportunities and threats presented by the external environment and the competition.

The factors are further sorted in accordance with their dual positive aspects (Strengths and opportunities) and dual negative aspects (Weaknesses and threats)

SWOT analysis isolates the key issues that will be important to the future of the organization and the subsequent marketing plan.

Marketing Objectives

With the results of the audit available, the active part of the marketing planning process begins. This stage in marketing planning is indeed the crux of the whole marketing process. The marketing objectives state where the company intends to be at some specific time in the future.

Marketing objective is essentially about the match between products and markets what products or services will be in what position in what markets. Pricing, distribution and advertising objectives are at a lower level and should not be confused with marketing objectives although they are part of the marketing strategy needed to achieve marketing objectives.

To be effective, objectives should be measurable. This measurement may be in terms of sales volume, money value, market share, or percentage penetration of distribution outlets. As it is measured, it can, within limits, be unequally monitored and corrective action taken as necessary. Usually marketing objectives must be based above all on the organization financial objectives and financial measurement are converted into the related marketing measurements.

Marketing Strategies

A marketing strategy is essentially a pattern or plan that integrates an organizations major goals policies and action sequence in to a cohesive whole. It tells about how to achieve the goals or results or objectives are to be achieved. Marketing strategies are generally concerned with 4 **P**'s of marketing.

Product Strategies

a. Developing new products, repositioning or re-launching existing once, and scrapping old ones.
b. Adding new features and benefits.
c. Balancing product portfolios.
d. Changing the design or packaging.

Pricing Strategies

a. Setting the price to skim or to penetrate.
b. Pricing for different market segments.
c. Deciding how to meet competitive pricing.

Promotional Strategies

a. Specifying the advertising platform and media.
b. Public relation strategies.

c. Organizations the sales force to cover new products and services or markets.

Place Strategies

a. Choosing the channels.
b. Deciding customer service levels.

Marketing Plans and Programmes

Next step in the marketing planning process is to develop the overall marketing strategies into detailed plans and programmes. Although these detailed plans may cover each of the four P's the focus will vary depending on the organizations specific strategies. A product oriented company will focus its plans for the four Ps around each of its products. A market or geographically oriented company will concentrate on each market or geographical area. Each will base its plans on the detailed needs of its customers and on the strategies chosen to satisfy these needs. The plans should be:

1. **Clear:** They should be an unambiguous statement of exactly what is to be done.
2. **Quantified:** The predicted outcome of each activity should be quantified so that its performance can be monitored.
3. **Focused:** They should be focused.
4. **Realistic:** They should be achievable.
5. **Agreed upon:** Managers responsible to implement the plan should be committed to them and agree that they are achievable.

Marketing Plan Structure

The marketing plan should be formalized as a written document and might contain the following sections.

1. Mission statement.
2. Summary of performance including reasons for good or bad performance.
3. Summary of three years financial projections.
4. Market overview.
5. SWOT analysis of major projects/markets.
6. Portfolio summary (a summary of SWOT's).
7. Assumptions.

8. Setting objectives.
9. Detailed financial projections for three years.

Marketing Budgets

The classic quantification of a marketing plan appears in the form of budgets. Because these are so rigorously quantified, they are particularly important. They should, thus, represent an unequivocal projection of actions and expected results. What is more, they should be capable of being monitored accurately; and, indeed, performance against budget is the main (regular) management review process.

The purpose of a marketing budget is, thus, to pull together all the revenues and costs involved in marketing into one comprehensive document. It is a managerial tool that balances what is needed to be spent against what can be afforded, and helps make choices about priorities. It is then used in monitoring performance in practice.

The marketing budget is usually the most powerful tool by which you think through the relationship between desired results and available means. Its starting point should be the marketing strategies and plans, which have already been formulated in the marketing plan itself; although, in practice, the two will run in parallel and will interact. At the very least, the rigorous, highly quantified, budgets may cause a rethink of some of the more optimistic elements of the plans.

As mentioned in the previous paragraphs quantification of marketing plan appears in the form of budgets. The purpose of marketing budget is to pull all the revenues and costs involved in marketing together into one comprehensive document. Managers can choose some of the following budgeting approaches.

1. **Affordability:** As per affordability method a reasonable budget what can be afforded by the organization is decided upon. This figure is most often based on historical spending.
2. **Percentage of revenue:** In this approach budget will be set at a certain percentage of revenue, and this follows trends in sales.
3. **Competitive parity:** According to competitive parity method the organization fixes its budgets as per the competitors spending.
4. **Zero based budgeting:** This approach considers the marketing plan objectives, together with the resulting planned activities, and prepares the budget.

Many organizations consider affordability and percentage of revenue methods to be realistic as it reflect the reality of the business strategies.

Measurement of Progress

The final stage of any marketing planning process is to establish targets (or standards) so that progress can be monitored. Accordingly, it is important to put both quantities and timescales into the marketing objectives (for example, to capture 20% by value of the market within two years) and into the corresponding strategies.

Changes in the environment mean that the forecasts often have to be changed. Along with these, the related plans may well also need to be changed. Continuous monitoring of performance, against predetermined targets, represents a most important aspect of this. However, perhaps even more important is the enforced discipline of a regular formal review. Again, as with forecasts, in many cases the best (most realistic) planning cycle will revolve around a quarterly review. Best of all, at least in terms of the quantifiable aspects of the plans, if not the wealth of backing detail, is probably a quarterly rolling review-planning one full year ahead each new quarter. Of course, this does absorb more planning resource; but it also ensures that the plans embody the latest information, and - with attention focused on them so regularly - forces both the plans and their implementation to be realistic.

Plans only have validity if they are actually used to control the progress of a company: Their success lies in their implementation, not in the writing.

Performance Analysis

The most important elements of marketing performance, which are normally tracked, are:

1. *Sales analysis:* Most organizations track their sales results; or, in non-profit organizations for example, the number of clients. The more sophisticated track them in terms of 'sales variance'—the deviation from the target figures—which allows a more immediate picture of deviations to become evident. 'Micro-analysis', investigates detailed problems, then investigates the

individual elements (individual products, sales territories, customers and so on) which are failing to meet targets.

2. *Market share analysis:* Few organizations track market share though it is often an important metric. Though absolute sales might grow in an expanding market, a firm's share of the market can decrease which bodes ill for future sales when the market starts to drop. Where such market share is tracked, there may be a number of aspects which will be followed:
   - Overall market share.
   - Segment share in the specific targeted segment.
   - Relative share in relation to the market leaders.
   - Annual fluctuation rate of market share.
3. *Expense analysis:* The key ratio to watch in this area is usually the 'marketing expense to sales ratio'; although this may be broken down into other elements (advertising to sales, sales administration to sales, and so on).
4. *Financial analysis:* The 'bottom line' of marketing activities should at least in theory, be the net profit (for all except non-profit organizations, where the comparable emphasis may be on remaining within budgeted costs). There are a number of separate performance figures and key ratios which need to be tracked:
   - Gross contribution: Net profit
   - Gross profit: Return on investment
   - Net contribution: Profit on sales.

There can be considerable benefit in comparing these figures with those achieved by other organizations, especially those in the same industry. The most sophisticated use of this approach, however, is typically by those making use of PIMS (Profit Impact of Management Strategies), which was initiated by the General Electric Company and then developed by Harvard Business School, but now run by the Strategic Planning Institute.

The above performance analysis concentrate on the quantitative measures that are directly related to short term performance. However, there are a number of indirect measures tracking customer attitudes that can also indicate the organizations performance in terms of its long term marketing strengths and may accordingly be even more important indicators seem useful measures are the following:

1. **Market research** including customer panels.
2. **Lost business**—The orders that were lost because for example—the stock was not available or the product did not meet the customer's exact requirements.
3. **Customer complaints**—How many customers complain about the products services or the organization itself and what they complain about.

Relationship Analysis

Today relationship marketing has become vital for an organisation's long term success since it costs five times more to get a new customer than to keep a current one. Clearly companies that value commitment and trust relationships believes in relationship analysis. Organisations are keen in understanding customer expectations, building service partnership with customers, empowering employees and implementing total quality management. Relationship analysis measures customer satisfaction, customer loyalty, customer's perception of product and service quality and profitability.

BUSINESS ENVIRONMENT AND MARKETING

Most of the organizations devote immense efforts to optimizing the internal factors that are within their control. However, firms also need to be aware of their external environment and its current and potential effects. Any changes in the business environment, whether at home or abroad may have serious repercussions on the marketing activities of the firm. Managers must spend an increasing amount of their time to closely scrutinize factors which are external to the firm like societal factors, cultural factors, demographic factors, technological factors, economic factors, political factors and legal factors and try to understand their effects on the company. In addition, the marketer should develop an in-depth understanding of the position, motivation and capabilities of competing organizations as well as these organizations's response to the actions of other firms. All these knowledge is then used to develop competitive strategies that allow the firm to strengthen its position in the market.

The Technological Environment

The impact of changing technology is another major factor in the external environment. The rapid growth of fax machines, cellular telephones and modems demonstrates the revolution of unrestricted communication flows. Data communications are exploding propelled by the internet and the rapid convergence of data and video with traditional voice traffic. Concurrently the availability of information to be communicated is increasing dramatically. Since all this information includes details about lifestyles, opportunities and aspirations, the implications of this technology revolution for marketers are major. A growing global awareness of products is likely to ease international product introductions, and such greater ease will also encourage the emergence of greater global competition for market share both at home and abroad.

The impact of information technology on business and marketing are huge and the use of electronic data interchange, merchandise scanning, and increased data sharing is restructuring the ways firms do business. Technology affects the entire marketing strategy framework and covers the relationships with suppliers and manufactures, the internal organization of the firm, and the firm's interaction with inputs customers. Even though the technology has been available for some time we are entering new era in terms of its applications. The tools and connectivity of the digital age now give a way to easily obtain, share and act on information in new and remarkable ways. All kinds of information, numbers, text, sound, and video can be put into the digital form that any computer can store, process, and forward. Standard hardware combined with standard software platform has created economies of scale that make powerful computing solutions available inexpensively to companies of all sizes. And the personal computer means that individual knowledge workers have a powerful tool for analyzing and using the information delivered by these solutions. Because much of marketing is a dialogue, and information technology both enhances and restructures the existing forms of communication markets will be affected by information innovations more than even before.

Technology also permits marketers to work with their customers in more efficient ways. By linking purchase with specific customers, marketers can develop promotional programmes based on specific purchase behaviour. Information provides greater transparency of the market and enhances the customer's ability to make better decisions.

Information technology also brings major effects on the internal operations of firms like major reduction of total stocks at its distribution centres, lead times of one to two days on fresh foods, out of stock conditions reduced by 30%, reduction of storage space from 40 to 20% of total store floor space and productivity benefits which runs to million of rupees.

The Economic Environment

The marketer is affected by economic factors, primarily globalization, regional economic integration, and exchange rates. World markets are today more intertwined than ever before due to globalization. Marketers must therefore broaden their horizons when looking at market opportunities and threats. A firm's customer base is no longer restricted to the home country, but can be found around the world, likewise competition does nor emanate only from established domestic competitors, but can appear overnight from foreign shores.

Regional economic integration is another major phenomenon affecting the marketer. Increasingly countries engage in economic cooperation to use their respective resources more efficiently and to provide larger markets for member country producers. Global integration has successfully reduced red tape, documentation hassles, and transportation difficulties. Harmonizations of rules and standards have made the achievement of economics of scale easier. By reducing barriers between markets, such integration has also increased the levels of efficiency and competition.

The economic environment has also been greatly affected by the powerful effects of exchange rate. Rapid changes in currency value have a major effect on the marketer, particularly when doing business internationally. Long-term strategic plans can be ruined if major shifts in exchange rates occur.

The Political and Legal Environment

Politics and laws play a critical role in marketing. Even the best laid plans can go awry as a result of unexpected political or legal influences. The failure to anticipate these factors can be disastrous to even a successful venture. Governments affect firms through their legislations and regulations which might specify anything from the ingredient used in their products to the buildings in which their employees may work. Interest groups can put pressure on firms and alter corporate activities by shaping selective dimensions of the way the public sees the firm.

Many laws and regulation may not be designed specifically to address marketing issues, yet they can have a major impact on a firm's opportunity. For instance, cost of adhering to safety regulations significantly affects the pricing policies of firms. Intellectual property rights legislation and the extent of its enforcement may either allow a firm to recoup its investment into innovation or deprive it of its rightful returns, thereby determining the firm's ability to invest in further research and development to create new products. In addition firms are often affected by administrative regulations that are developed by agencies in order to implement broader laws particularly in the international area.

Most aspects of marketing transitions are covered by one or another form of legislations and at least by law of contract. The marketing manager must be aware of the legal aspects that directly affect the firm and these effects vary form industry to industry and form country to country. The chemical industry for instance is driven by legislation on safety.

Political action is not confined just to government and legislatures. It can result from interest groups as well. Pressure groups campaign often to change legislation but also work to change the public's awareness and buying habits. Interest groups are an influential force in the external environment. Often able to garner support very quickly, special interest groups can have a dramatic impact on the company's marketing efforts.

The increasing scale of the discontinuous changes means that marketers must be ever more sensitive to these potential, dramatic shifts in the environment. They must also develop the ability, based on adequate resources and prior planning, to cope with such changes.

For instance—is there any connection between Beijing Olympics 2008 and price increase of medicines in India? Yes, it seems, according to pharmaceutical manufacturers. The price of many medicines has increased much before Olympics commenced in September 2008. The price increase is between 30 to 100%.

The reason behind this is quiet surprising. As everybody knows the tablets and capsules are covered/ packed by/with strips. Major chunk of strips are sourced from China, as the production cost of strips in china are comparatively less. The government of China, in the wake of Olympics, to avoid environmental pollution, has strictly controlled the production of strips. So the production of strips has almost completely stopped and it resulted shortage of strips and even shortage of medicines and the outcome is price increase.

Here a question may arise. As there is price control on medicines in India how does it affect the general public? In fact in India price control is only on 80 medicines. This is only 20% of the total medicines sold in the market. The rest 80% of medicines manufactured by domestic and multinational companies are sold in the market without any price control, or in other words these companies are free to fix the prices. To make matters worse many medicines which come under price control are not manufactured by pharma companies citing the reason that they are not profitable.

Environmental Analysis

To cope with all the changes in its external environment the firm must first discover what opportunities and threats this environment holds for the organizations this process requires an environmental analysis. Three main mechanisms that serve to conduct such an analysis are environmental scanning, Delphi studies and scenario building.

Competition

Competition is a major factor in most markets. The marketer must therefore understand the relative performance of his or her offering when compared to the competition. Only with an in-depth understanding of the competition is it possible to formulate competitive strategies that permit the firm to prevail in the fierce battle for resources. The first level of the competitive environment is the industry within which the organization operates. The organization should be well aware of competitive structure, competitive response (Non-response or slow response, fast response and focused response), competitive strategies, etc. for survival and growth.

Marketing Research and Marketing Intelligence System

The tool for listening to customers is marketing research. Marketing research also assists managers in decision making. Marketers are often faced with a lack of information and therefore with uncertanity. Marketing research requires a constant flow of information, which typically covers markets, customers and consumers, competitive activities, the impact of environmental factors and the organization's own marketing activities. As a result of the widening availability of computerized databases the process of collecting and distributing marketing information has become systematized. The system that handles these processes in a controlled and coordinated fashion has come to be called that marketing intelligence system. Such a system collects and organizes data that are relevant to the marketer in terms of planning implementation.

Two types of external data are available to the marketer. These are secondary data and primary data both available outside the firm The main source of external data is usually published data often referred to as secondary data because they have been generated in response to someone else's questions. Finding secondary data is the key to sound research. Libraries, directories and newsletters, commercial information providers, trade associations, electronic information providers, etc. are major sources of secondary data. Source quality, data quality and data compatibility are important considerations when collecting secondary data.

Primary data is collected from consumers or customers usually on a sample basis. Primary data is collected through mail, telephone and personal interviewing. Retail audits, panel research and omnibus surveys are common methods used in primary research.

MARKET DEMAND

Key precursor to marketing planning is market demand forecasting. With business environments changing rapidly, it is no longer possible to repeat the actions that have worked in the past. Most organizations face a degree of uncertainty. The more uncertainty, greater is the risk to the organization. The primary task of market demand forecasting is to reduce uncertainity to the possible lowest level. Another task of market forecasting is to identify and quantify organizational environmental changes. This will provide the organization to identify threats and opportunities.

Depending on the time span there are three types of forecasts - short term, medium term and long term forecasts. Short term forecast are tactical in nature. They are done for a month or a quarter, as input to the normal business planning and control processes. Short term forecast are also used for production scheduling, information transmission and control. Medium term forecasting are done annually and is done as the main input for the budget planning processes. Long-term forecast is typically for five years. Strategic decisions, resource planning and communication are the major decisions associated with long term forecasting.

Forecasting techniques can be categorized into qualitative methods and quantitative methods. Individual or expert opinions, expert panel method, technological forecasting, decision tree, scenario are the common qualitative methods of forecasting techniques. Qualitative methods are usually used for long-term forecasting. Most of the mathematical techniques like period actuals and percentage changes, exponential smoothing, advanced time – series analysis and models, multiple regression analysis, econometric models, spreadsheets, etc. falls under quantitative forecasting techniques, which is short term in nature.

The prescription drug industry is affected by the basic characteristics of supply and demand, as are other industries. In general, supply and demand are affected by many economic, social, and environmental factors. The characteristics of the goods themselves, the nature of the sales outlet, the socioeconomic status of the buyer, and the availability of other goods and alternate sources of supply are a few of the factors that may affect supply. However, drugs are somewhat peculiar in that the demand may be affected to a considerable degree by the influence of third and even fourth parties to the traditional buyer-seller relationship. The most frequently discussed relationship in the supply demand interface is that between price and quantity.

Inelasticity of demand commonly exists in the prescription drug industry. Changes in price of prescription drugs do not normally result in proportionate inverse changes in the quantity demanded. The nature of the pharmaceutical product itself is the primary reason of its inelasticity. Prescription drugs are necessary to health and within reasonable limits will be purchased in spite of price increases. Furthermore, there is little reason for purchasing more of a drug than is needed regardless of how much the price decreases. Apart from the nature of the product at least two other factors contribute to price inelasticity. The physician's role as the decision maker in the choice of prescription drugs tends to make price a secondary consideration. Moreover, the efforts of the pharmaceutical industry toward product differentiation, either through promotion or actual product changes, reduce the importance of price as a consideration in drug choice and consequently reduce the elasticity of demand.

The quantity demanded may be affected significantly by seasonal variations. Production and marketing planning are influenced by seasonal variations. Both production and marketing planning depends upon accurate forecasting of seasonal change in quantity demanded for individual products. From the production point of view this is important for scheduling and purchasing. In marketing, sales quotas and plans, advertising campaigns, and budgets are all factors that are significantly affected by seasonal patterns. For instance pharmaceutical products for fever and cold are sold in larger quantities during the winter months, cardiovascular drugs are sold more during seasons of extreme temperatures as extreme temperature affect the heart patient and his consequent use of medication. As well dermatologic drugs and anti-allergic drugs are sold in large quantities during the summer months because of the increased exposure to allergy-aggravating substances during this period of outdoor living.

Pharmaceutical Marketing

3

Pharmaceutical marketing which is a subspecialty of marketing encompasses all the activities carried out by various individuals or organizations to actualize markets for pharmaceutical care. The emphasis of pharmaceutical marketing is on pharmaceutical care rather than pharmaceutical drugs. In other words the focus of pharmaceutical marketing is on the patient, not on manufacturers, chemists, etc. At the same time all the participants in providing pharmaceutical care to the patient such as pharmaceutical manufacturers, wholesalers, chemists, doctors or physicians, hospital pharmacies, insurance companies, warehousing and transportation companies, etc. are actively involved in pharmaceutical marketing.

Marketing of pharmaceutical products can be described as providing the right drug at the right price, at the right place, with the right information, to the right market. This will ensure achieving the marketing objectives as well as the overall organisational objective. Pharmaceutical companies can achieve its marketing objectives by prudent marketing management through following steps:

1. Formulation of marketing objectives
2. Market opportunity assessment
3. Resource and environment analysis
4. Market segmentation
5. Identification of target markets
6. Developing optimal marketing mix
7. Marketing control and evaluation.

The pharmaceutical market is unique in the importance of the influence of a non-purchaser on the purchasing habits of the ultimate consumer. So it becomes necessary to classify physicians as thoroughly as the patients. A further peculiarity of the pharmaceutical market is the importance of the disease entity. Incidence of disease is an important classificatory device for identifying and quantifying a market for pharmaceutical products especially prescription drugs.

PHARMACEUTICAL MARKET AND MARKETING RESEARCH

Traditionally a 'Market' was a physical place where buyers and sellers gathered to buy and sell goods. Economists describe a market as a collection of buyers and sellers who transact over a particular product or product class like pharmaceutical market. Modern economics abound in such markets. Manufacturers go to resource markets (raw material markets, labor markets, money marketers), buy resources and turn them into good and services, and then sell finished products to intermediaries, who sell them to consumers. Consumers sell their labour and receive money with which they pay for goods and services. The government collects tax revenues to buy goods and services to provide public services. Each nation's economy and the global economy consist of complex interacting set of markets linked through exchange process.

On the contrary, MARKET often uses the term market to cover various groupings of customers. They view sellers as constituting the industry and the buyers as constituting the MARKET. They talk about need markets (the diet seeking market), product markets (the pharmaceutical market), demographic market (the youth market), the geographic market (the Asian market) etc. There lies a strong relationship between the industry and the market. Sellers and buyers are connected by four flows. The sellers send goods and services and communications (ads, direct mail) to the market, in return they receive money and information (attitudes, sales data). In short there is an exchange of money for goods and services and an exchange of information to the industry from the market.

So industry is a collection of sellers and market is a collection of buyers. Pharmaceutical market is nothing but a collection of buyers who has an interest to purchase pharmaceutical products. In other words pharmaceutical market comprises of all customers who have needs that may be fulfilled by the pharmaceutical companies offerings. Pharmaceutical market may also referred as the prescription market, the hospital market, the antibiotic market, etc.

Pharmaceutical companies find that the markets that they serve are dynamic with customers, competitions and market conditions continually changing. And marketing efforts that can work today cannot be relied upon to be successful in the future. Meeting changing conditions require pharmaceutical marketers have sufficient market knowledge in order to make the right adjustments in the marketing strategies. For pharma marketers gaining knowledge is accomplished through marketing research or market research.

Many feel that there is a difference between marketing research and market research. They opinion that marketing research covers a broader array of research efforts associated with marketing desicions, while market research is specific in understanding nuances of a particular market.

Marketing research: It is the systematic and objective identification, collection, analysis, and dissemination of information for the purpose of assisting management in decision making related to the identification and solution of problems and opportunities in marketing. The goal of marketing research is to identify and assess how changing elements of the marketing mix impacts customer behaviour.

Market research: It is broader in scope and examines all aspects of a business environment. It asks questions about competitors, market structure, government regulations, economic trends, technological advances, and numerous other factors that make up the business environment. Sometimes the term refers more particularly to the financial analysis of companies, industries, or sectors. In this case, financial analysts usually carry out the research and provide the results to investment advisors and potential investors.

Role of Marketing Research

The task of pharmaceutical marketing research is to provide management with relevant, accurate, reliable, valid, and current information. Competitive marketing environment and the ever-increasing costs attributed to poor decision making require that marketing research provide sound information. Sound decisions are not based on gut feeling, intuition, or even pure judgment.

Marketing managers make numerous strategic and tactical decisions in the process of identifying and satisfying customer needs. They make decisions about potential opportunities, target market selection, market segmentation, planning and implementing marketing programmes, marketing performance, and control. These decisions are complicated by interactions between the controllable marketing variables of product, pricing, promotion, and distribution. Further complications are added by uncontrollable environmental factors such as general economic conditions, technology, public policies and laws, political environment, competition, and social and cultural changes. Another factor in this mix is the complexity of consumers. Marketing research helps the marketing manager link the marketing variables with the environment and the consumers. It helps remove some of the uncertainty by providing relevant information about the marketing variables, environment, and consumers. In the absence of relevant information, consumers' response to marketing programmes cannot be predicted reliably or accurately. Ongoing marketing research programmes provide information on controllable and non-controllable factors and consumers; this information enhances the effectiveness of decisions made by marketing managers.

Traditionally, marketing researchers were responsible for providing the relevant information and marketing decisions were made by the managers. However, the roles are changing and marketing researchers are becoming more involved in decision making, whereas marketing managers are becoming more involved with research. The role of marketing research in managerial decision making is explained further using the framework of the **DECIDE** model:

D - Define the marketing problem
E - Enumerate the controllable and uncontrollable decision factors
C - Collect relevant information
I - Identify the best alternative
D - Develop and implement a marketing plan
E - Evaluate the decision and the decision process.

The **DECIDE** *model* conceptualizes managerial decision making as a series of six steps. The decision process begins by precisely defining the problem or opportunity, along with the objectives and constraints. Next, the possible decision factors that make up the alternative courses of action (controllable factors) and uncertainties (uncontrollable factors) are enumerated. Then, relevant information on the alternatives and possible outcomes is collected. The next step is to select the best alternative based on chosen criteria or measures of success. Then a detailed plan to implement the alternative selected is developed and put into effect. Last, the outcome of the decision and the decision process itself are evaluated.

Characteristics of Marketing Research

Marketing Research is Systematic

Thus systematic planning is required at all the stages of the marketing research process. The procedures followed at each stage are methodologically sound, well documented, and, as much as possible, planned in advance. Marketing research uses the scientific method in that data are collected and analyzed to test prior notions or hypotheses.

Marketing Research is Objective

It attempts to provide accurate information that reflects a true state of affairs. It should be conducted impartially. While research is always influenced by the researcher's research philosophy, it should be free from the personal or political biases of the researcher or the management. Research which is motivated by personal or political gain involves a breach of professional standards. Such research is deliberately biased so as to result in predetermined findings. The motto of every researcher should be, "Find it and tell it like it is". The objective nature of marketing research underscores the importance of ethical considerations, which are discussed later in the chapter.

Marketing Research

Involves the *identification,* collection, analysis, *and dissemination of information:* Each phase of this process is important. We identify or define the marketing research problem or opportunity and then determine what information is needed to investigate it and inferences are drawn. Finally, the findings, implications and recommendations are provided in a format that allows the information to be used for management decision making and to be acted upon directly. It should be emphasized that marketing research is conducted to assist management in decision making and is not: A means or an end in itself.

Measuring the Market

The measurement of product movement at the final point of sale in the long distribution line is a fundamental function of marketing research. Measurement may be the number of times an item is sold, the number of units of an item that have been sold, or the value of the total sales from one period to another. The aggregate figures for all similar products measure individual product fields and the combination of all fields yields the measurement of a market. The following figures can be computed from these data.

1. The size of pharmaceutical market expressed in numbers of transactions of individual sales, total units or rupees.
2. Growth or decline trends of total pharmaceutical markets, individual field, individual products, and product forms.
3. Regional or geographic variations in markets.
4. Time series analysis – secular trend, cyclical variation, seasonal pattern, and episodic movement.
5. Singular, partial or multiple correlations with other series of factors.

Pharmaceutical industry is considered as one of the most "data rich" of all industries. As a result it uses maximum market and marketing research information. To a large degree, this wealth of data regarding the pharmaceutical marketplace is a function of the many inherently unique aspects of the pharmaceutical marketing process.

Pharmaceutical companies produce and market two types of products, i.e. the prescription product that may be obtained by consumers only with a doctors prescription and the over the-counter product that may be purchased without a prescription. Though there is a growth in the over-the-counter pharmaceutical market in recent years, most of the fundamental business of pharmaceutical companies still remains the production and marketing of prescription drugs. Pharmaceutical industry is unique in that it does not market its products to the ultimate consumer, the patient, but instead to an intermediary, the physician or other licensed prescribes. Though the patient is the ultimate customer the physician is the decision maker in pharmaceutical marketing. As mentioned above pharmaceutical marketing is unique due to the reasons given in the following paragraphs.

a. For a pharmaceutical company the target market is the population of licensed prescribes in the country, rather than the consumers of the products. Another target of the marketing effort for prescription drugs can be considered as the licensed pharmacists in the country, because some times they decide with regard to the specific brand of drug to be dispensed to the patient. Here too, however, the focus is on an intermediary rather than on the ultimate consumer.
b. The selling of prescription drugs to the end user is restricted to the comparatively small numbers of pharmacists and pharmacies in the country rather than to the substantially larger number of retailers and retail outlets that would normally be the case for a consumer product, because to store and sell prescription drugs one need a license.
c. A record of every transaction involving the sale or dispensing of a prescription drug to the consumer is created and maintained with the doctor and the pharmacist which is being specific to the patient, physician, pharmacy, and product as purchase of prescription drugs by consumers requires the presentation of authorization by a licensed prescribe in the form of a written prescription.

These unique aspects of prescription product marketing, are of considerable importance in Pharmaceutical marketing/market research. There is virtually no difficulty in finding physicians, pharmacists, pharmacies, or hospitals because product choice decisions and product movement in the multicrore rupees prescription drug industry are represented by a relatively small population of licensed prescribers, retail pharmacies and hospital pharmacies as compared to crores of customers and equal number of decision makers, and lakhs of retail outlets as in the case of marketing and selling of other consumer products. Hardly any records are maintained either by manufacturer or retailer regarding their customers in other consumer products. Only overall sales data will be available.

d. As well as the degree of error in pharmaceutical market data is also negligible because information on the physician's type of practice, specialty, year graduated from medical school, medical school attended, and location of practice and information about retail pharmacies in terms of their type, size, and location and information's about hospitals, type, bed size, affiliation with learning institutions, equipment available are either readily available or easy to find out.

e. As physicians who are the intermediaries in pharmaceutical marketing have received the same basic and professional education there is fair amount of homogeneity in prescription behaviour which facilitates the conduct of pharmaceutical market research. This is the case with pharmacists too. Due to the homogeneity factor no wide variations from physician to physician are found in terms of socioeconomic considerations. Most participants in the health care area are professionals and tend to communicate on an inter and intra group basis better than the average consumer does with other consumers. Similarity in thinking and activity among the members of a particular group generally tends to facilitate researching of the group.

f. Pharmaceutical market research in the prescription drug segment is somewhat easier because most of the decisions made by customers/prescribers (doctors) in the market are based on knowledge. The decisions are rational in nature and not emotional.

g. As mentioned earlier in pharmaceutical market research, the researcher does not have to create or search extensively for records of fact regarding decision or activity because records are required to be maintained about every transaction regarding the sale of a prescription-drug to a consumer.

All the above mentioned reasons have made pharmaceutical market research especially the prescription drug market research much easier, less complicated and hassle free in terms of identifying information sources, searching for information, culling out information or data, for the marketing researchers. This is not the case in other consumer goods market research. This is certainly a major reason for the data rich pharmaceutical industry.

PHARMACEUTICAL MARKETING RESEARCH (AUDIT) ACTIVITIES

The major research (audit) activities conducted in pharmaceutical market research are:

1. Retail pharmacy purchase audit.
2. Hospital purchase audit.
3. Warehouse withdrawal audit.
4. Retail pharmacy prescription audit.
5. Physician panels
6. Promotional media audit.
7. Retail sales audit.

Retail Pharmacy Purchase Audit

Retail pharmacy purchase audit measures the flow of product either directly from a manufacturer or from a wholesaler into retail pharmacies. So it also known as "inflow" audit. The purchase audits reflect all purchases by a pharmacy or hospital whether or not they were purchased directly from a manufacturer or from a wholesaler.

Warehouse Withdrawal Audit

Warehouse withdrawal audit measures the withdrawal of pharmaceutical products from the pharmaceutical wholesaler and from major drug chain warehouses. Though there are lots of similarities between retail pharmacy purchase audit and ware house withdrawal audit the main difference is that the warehouse withdrawal audit focuses on the warehouse segment only and purchases directly from the manufacturer are not represented in the auditing process.

Retail Pharmacy Prescription Audits

Retail pharmacy prescription audit measures the outflow of prescription drugs from the pharmacy to the consumer. Prescription audit data are the most sensitive indicators of prescription product performance in the marketplace. Prescriptions are indicators of what is presently occurring in terms of demand. Prescription audit provides information about changes in prescribing patterns, which ultimately will affect demand and sales of the pharmaceutical product. Prescription data are also viewed by most pharmaceutical marketers as the best indicators of the outcome of marketing or promotional efforts to create new business. New prescriptions for a product, however, are a reasonably good indicator of the trend in generating new patient business for the product.

Retail Sales Audit

Retail sales audit is primarily used to measure sales of non-prescription drugs. One type of retail sales audit may be described as "opening inventory plus delivered purchases minus ending inventory." Mainly because of time and cost considerations, this type of audit is conducted for selected products of interest to the subscriber as opposed to the "all products, all categories" approach most of the audit services already described.

Data Processing, Data Analysis and Interpretation

Once the data has been collected the process of analysis begins. But almost invariably the data must first be translated into a form appropriate for analysis. Raw data as they are received from the field in primary data collection, are in no condition for interpretation. Such data constitute bits of information recorded on many individual forms, and substantial work must be done on them. Therefore, the bits of raw data must be transformed into information that will answer the market research objective. The decisions made about these preparatory steps are based on assumptions involving general logic about the interpretive process and about the supposed nature of the data relative to the appropriate analysis.

The transformations of raw data into useful information requires that the data be validated, edited, coded and keypunched so that it may be transferred to a computer or any other data storage device. If the amount of data gathered is large then there are many advantages in utilizing a computer for data processing.

Until the late eighties, mostly manual methods were used in India for data processing. But now it is rarely done manually. In almost all cases computers are used. Software packages like SPSS, SAS, STATISTICA, SYSTAT, etc. are the most common packages available in India for data processing.

One limitation of doing analysis on the computer with these statistical packages is that all data must be converted into numerical form. Otherwise, it cannot be counted or manipulated for analysis. So all the data must be coded and converted to numbers, if it is non-numerical. Using, nominal scale variables (categorical variables) need to be coded and entered into the packages. An important aspect of coding is to remember which code stands for what. Most software packages have a facility called definition of value labels for each variable, which should be used to define the codes for every value of a variable.

Having gathered the data from primary sources the researcher proceeds toward the drawing of conclusions by logical inferences, i.e. the data has to be analyzed. Analysis of data is the process by which data is converted into useful information. At this stage those data are only hundreds or thousands of responses or observations, incapable of interpretation until converted into significant statistical information. Statistical analysis is the refinement and manipulation of data that prepared them for the application of logical inference. Broadly we can classify analysis into three types:

1. Univeriate, involving a single variable at a time,
2. Bivariate, involving two variables at a time
3. Multivariate, involving three or more variables simultaneously

The choice of which of the above types of data analysis to use depends on at least three factors:

1. The scale of measurement of the data
2. The research design and
3. Assumptions about the test statistic being used.

There are three chief phases in data analyzes

1. Bringing the raw data into measured order data (arrays, tabulations, establishing categories, percentages, etc.).
2. Summarizing the data (statistical summarization – measures of central tendency and dispersion, graphical presentations).
3. Applying analytical methods to manipulate the data so that their interrelationships and quantitative meanings become evident. (Examining difference, analyze experimental data, investigate associations).

It was mentioned earlier about the general data processing applications of statistical packages. But this is not all that these packages are capable of. They can help us to do a lot of statistical tests, like the Chi-squared, the t-test and the F-test. They can also be used to perform analysis such as correlation and regression analysis, ANOVA or analysis of variance, factor analysis, cluster analysis, discriminanat analysis, multidimensional scaling, conjoint analysis, and many other advanced statistical analysis. The packages like SPSS. SAS, SYSTAT generally perform most of these analyses. In addition the statistical packages also have varying graphical capabilities for drawing graphs. Some of the packages require a large amount of computer memory to operate some of the advanced multivariate statistical techniques, particularly if the data size is large.

Interpretation means to bring out the meaning of data or it means to convert mere data into information. The climax of the research process is approached as one prepared to draw conclusions from the data analyzed. The whole investigation culminates and reaches fruition in drawing inferences that lead to conclusions as to the course of action or problem solution. This phase calls for a high degree of interpretive skill, both quantitative and logical: (a) Induction and (b) deduction are two phases of logical thought used in drawing inferences from data. Logicians distinguish between inductive reasoning.

Pharmaceutical market research encompasses the following activities:

1. Data base creation
2. Text mining
3. Web mining
4. Numerical data mining.

Data Base Creation

Biomedical research including genomics and proteomics has made tremendous progress in generating new insights for drug discovery. The knowledge thus obtained should be maintained in databases which will allow analyzing large volumes of data. This requires in-depth database research and technology development to with hold the ever-growing volumes of data. In the chemistry front, relational chemical databases for the molecules of specific interest obtained through manual literature curation have gained importance. The ability to search based on substructure/similarity searching methodologies provides ease in usage. Database development solutions integrate the tools developed for Data mining. This especially helps in the analysis of published text data and storing into the database for complex queries. Through the innovative workflow concepts of typical drug discovery organizations, the different data are connected for varied queries. An intelligent query system coupled with the database would be ideal for obtaining the end users compliance. Thus a step towards development of customized databases with flexible data storage and data retrieval options would be appreciated for sure.

Text Mining

Data mining which includes text mining, web mining, and numerical data mining automates the process of finding relationships and patterns in raw data (text, web and numerical). It is used as an automated decision support system or assessed by a human analyst. The technologies involved are statistical calculations, neural networks, evolutionary programming, decision trees, genetic algorithms, nonlinear regression methods.

Extraction of knowledge from huge chunk of scientific literature poses a huge challenge to the informatics community. The prime suppository for biomedical literature "PUBMED" seems to grow with an extra million every three months. Pub Med having already crossed 16 million articles, the knowledge management has become an extremely crucial factor. For a researcher to equip with the updated and comprehensive information pertaining to his own research, it is necessary to develop systems that could easily fetch specific information in a quick time. Since the major chunk of literary information is in the form of unstructured text, an intelligent text mining system could provide a platform for extracting and managing specific information at the entity level. For example, information pertaining to genes, proteins, diseases, organisms, chemical substances, etc. It would also aid in providing insights into inter-relationships such as protein-protein, gene-gene, protein-chemical, gene-disease and drug-drug interactions.

Text mining can be applied to the following areas for data curation and database population in a semi-automated manner.

- Bio-medical literature (Pub med Central, Medline Abstracts)
- Chemical literature (ACS Publications)
- Patents (USPTO)
- Clinical documents (Clinical trial and research) and
- Other medical literary sources.

Web Mining

With the enormous growth of World Wide Web, the informational resource pertaining to biology and chemistry through internet have reached new heights. The heterogeneous platforms and data types spread across the internet makes it difficult to have easy access to an end user. Up-to-date there are more than 1000 web portals which provide access to various biological and chemical databases. Accessibility to these heterogeneous databases under one roof would be a formidable solution. To achieve this it requires customized search engines and indexing mechanisms which could map the URLs, web content and associated files to extract the static as well as the dynamic data. Thus a web mining technology could be the fore runner in providing online and instant solution for gathering information across the World Wide Web.

Numerical Data Mining

Automated and semi-automated systems for high throughput screening and analysis in drug research generate huge amount of numerical data. The interpretation of results from these numerical data involves normalization and identification of nominal patterns which in turn requires statistical techniques to be followed. This has to be addressed through the development of component and field specific applications. Likewise the chemical structures are now efficiently handled in the form of numbers and combinations. The properties and the structural configuration of chemical compounds are now manipulated in the form of numbers. Thus a major challenge is ahead in handling these numerical data. This issue could be addressed through techniques such as Clustering, Decision Trees and Neural Networks.

It may be noted that there are many organizations in India who conduct pharmaceutical research and analysis. There services can be out sourced by pharmaceutical companies, R&D units in Drug Discovery organizations of the Pharma/Biotech industry, Publicly funded Research Institutes and Universities and Larger Bio/ Cheminformatics companies, etc.

The common services provided by these organizations are Database Creation, Protein Annotation, Signal Processing Analysis, Signal Processing Tool Development, QSAR Analysis, Text Mining and Web Mining, etc.

The services offered to Bio and Cheminformatics companies are: Content curation services in Biology and Chemistry, customized biological/chemistry databases, Bio/Cheminformatics software development, Data analysis and visualization and statistical analysis tool development.

These organizations helps there clients in data analysis too. Large volumes of experimental data generated by scientists in the research units of organizations need sophisticated tools for analysis and arriving at meaningful information. They help pharmaceutical organizations in their research efforts either by providing specialized tools for analysis or by performing the data analysis for them. They discover various resources and integrate them to form experimental functionality using new tools. The end result is an analysis of immense potential and adaptability, useful to scientists.

By outsourcing knowledge-based processes pharmaceutical companies can save valuable amounts of time and money that can then be utilized in other important processes. They receive the standards of quality and efficiency that they are looking for and also have an expert's skill and professionalism. With growing competition among Research and Analysis service providers. Outsourcing is a best option to getting the most optimized results at an affordable price and utilizing your time to the maximum. O2I realizes that several companies are still apprehensive about sending confidential information to a company in another continent.

Pharmaceutical Research

India is considered an ideal research and analysis destination due to various favorable reasons.

With its firepower of engineers, chartered accountants, doctors, MBAs, lawyers, research analysts, scientific researchers and PhDs, India is well positioned to address the global Research and Analysis need with a focused array of Research and Analysis services. India provides ready access to a large intellectual pool with domain expertise in specialized areas, coupled with computer skills and proficiency in the English language, the ideal combination for successful offshore Research and Analysis.

India's higher education system: The Indian way of education which lays great emphasis on higher education and specialization, creates a readily available talent pool with specialized knowledge in any field. There is also tremendous emphasis on mathematics and science, resulting in a large number of science and engineering graduates.

The science and technology edge: The Government of India has set up IITs (Indian Institute of Technology) and IIMs (Indian Institute of Managements) across the country. These ivy-league institutes of formal education are centres of excellence competing with the best institutes worldwide. Another milestone was the establishment of IIIT (Indian Institute of Information Technology) as a joint initiative by the government and industry. Apart from producing BTech/MTech/PhD graduates, it also trains professionals and industry-sponsored candidates.

India has more than 250 universities (over 1200 colleges) and engineering colleges providing computer education at the degree/diploma level. The output of trained human power at the degree/diploma level has been consistently increasing since 1985. The formal education system is augmented by thousands of private training institutes providing computer education. There is also a large pool of MBAs.

With India's infotech sector firmly in a leadership position on the global map, its scientific and research talent has also been acknowledged by the world. India is an emerging hub for contract research and clinical trials. India's biotech sector spans the spectrum of Bio-Pharma, Bio-Agri, Bio-Industrial, Bio-informatics, and Bio-services industries. Renowned Indian scientific institutions provide high-quality R&D services to organizations worldwide. Among them are the Indian Institute of Science (IIS), the National Centre for Biological Sciences (NCBSs), Jawaharlal Nehru Centre for Advanced Scientific Research (JNCASR), Plant Genomics Center, New Delhi, Centre for Human Genetics, Bangalore, National Institute of Biological, New Delhi, Center for Cellular and Molecular

Biology (CCMB), Hyderabad, National Facility for Macromolecular Crystallography, BARC, Mumbai, National Facility for High Field NMR, TIFR, Mumbai Central Drug Research Institute, Lucknow, National Brain Research Center, New Delhi.

The english advantage: In all good educational institutions, from kindergarten to graduation and beyond, the preferred medium of education is English, resulting in a significantly large population of educated and qualified professionals with English language skills. Many of them think in English, write in English and speak English as if it were their mother tongue.

Government policies that aid outsourcing of research and analysis: The Indian government has recognized that knowledge processes will influence economic development extensively in the future and has taken remarkable measures towards liberalization and deregulation. Recent reforms have reduced licensing requirements, made foreign technology accessible, removed restrictions on investment and made the process of investment much easier. The government has been continuously improving infrastructure with better roads, setting up technology parks, opening up the telecom sector for enhanced connectivity, providing uninterrupted power to augment growth.

Knowledge parks: Global facilities in R&D infotech and biotech: The last five years have seen vast development in Knowledge Parks with infrastructure of global standards, in cities like Chennai, Bangalore and Gurgaon. Multi-tenanted 'intelligent' buildings, built-to-suit facilities, sprawling campuses are tailor-made to suit customer requirements. International Long Distance, National Long Distance and Basic Telephone services have been opened up for free competition. ISPs (Internet Service Providers) have been granted licenses freely to establish their own international gateways and submarine cable landing stations. Internet telephony too has been encouraged. Tax holidays and concessions for companies involved in scientific R&D are just some of the steps to create a pro-growth environment. Ernst and Young ranks India No.3 after Japan and Korea in the Asia Pacific Region in Biotechnology. There are five biotech parks in India. It will house the Institute of Bio-informatics and Applied Biotechnology, and the Centre for Human Genetics which will move there. The cream of the biotech companies in the growing pharma and agri-biotech sector will be invited to set up shop there.

India—The Trust Factor

Proactive measures are being taken to ensure that India is viewed as a destination for trustworthy outsourcing. Initiatives from individual companies to associations like NASSCOM (The National Association of Software Services Companies) and the Indian government, are working together to build trust in Brand India as the world's leading outsourcing centre and a growing Research and Analysis hub.

Data Privacy and Information Security Initiatives

The National Association of Software Services Companies (NASSCOM) collaborates with the government to ensure that India's data privacy legislation is aligned with those of the US. It also intends to have the security practices of all its 860 member companies audited by international accounting firms. The government has also taken initiatives to focus on the issues of data privacy, information security and Intellectual Property Rights (IPR). Indian companies are taking serious measures to protect the information of their customers. Common security procedures in companies ensure those employees' swipe identity cards through readers, have their bags and pockets searched, deposit cell phones, PDAs, pens and laptops in lockers, and shred notes of client conversations after the shift ends.

Employee Scrutiny

Companies have set up advanced systems to monitor phone conversations, guard data, and watch every move of their employees. Measures may also include biometric security checks such as retina scans and palm reading, to identify employees against their records. Employee background checks are a regular feature of the recruitment process. These measures work well towards alleviating concerns of privacy and information security of customers wishing to source services of Indian Research and Analysis Services vendors.

Bangalore, Hyderabad and Mumbai have been found to be low-risk outsourcing locations, in a recent study by Hill and Associates, an enterprise security and risk management consultancy firm.

Sustaining the Momentum

The Indian government has been taking the right steps to ensure an ever-increasing talent pool of highly qualified professionals. IITs/IIITs have been planned in every state. The industry would help formulate some of the courses offered to ensure that emerging professionals are in sync with industry requirements. There are plans to include computer courses in every engineering discipline in the country. So regardless of the discipline, every course in engineering, science and commerce should see the inclusion of computer science programmes. Existing premier institutions like the IITs, IISc, RECs (Regional Engineering Colleges) would be doubling or tripling their output by suitable restructuring.

Quality Initiatives

HRD divisions in most companies have well-defined processes to hire the right professionals. They allocate substantial energies towards regular training and constantly develop ways to address attrition. They have realized that the key to high-quality work output lies in the selection, hiring, training and retention of a skilled workforce.

Quality Standards

Companies in India have achieved high levels of quality standards. More than 200 companies are quality-accredited and serve over 255 Fortune 500 companies. India now has far more SEI CMM Level 5 companies than any other country. Many companies have aligned their Quality Management Systems with ISO 9000 standards.

The successful analysis and interpretation of marketing data, depends is contingent upon a number of factors. These factors are relevant whether the analyst is working with data reflecting a group of five physicians, or with data on the millions of transactions that are represented in the warehouse withdrawal audit.

Once a product is on the market, the main use of marketing data is to monitor the performance of a product across all the various aspects of the marketplace. Product sales, prescriptions, overall physician usage or by specialty or high prescribers, diagnosis, and location, for example, are all analyzed continuously to monitor progress of a product by itself as well as in relation to the market in which it competes. Invariably, this monitoring process reveals information that suggests the need for additional information or action, and the market or marketing research process takes another turn.

Drug Discovery and Drug Development

Drug discovery: It is the process by which potential drugs are discovered or designed. In the past most drugs have been discovered either by isolating the active ingredient from traditional remedies or by serendipitous discovery. Modern biotechnology often focuses on understanding the metabolic pathways related to a disease state or pathogen, and manipulating these pathways using molecular biology or Biochemistry. A great deal of early-stage drug discovery has traditionally been carried out by universities and research institutions.

Drug development: It is defined as the process of taking a new chemical lead through the stages necessary to allow it to be tested in human clinical trials. A broader definition defines drug development as the entire process of drug discovery and clinical testing of novel drug candidates.

After a product has been produced by chemical synthesis or isolation, compounds of interest are screened by pharmacologists using a sophisticated range of techniques, from sub-cellular particles to intact animals. Compounds with potential therapeutic applications are submitted for various toxicological examinations, including determinations of lethal doses in several species of animals and pathologic studies for detection of organ toxicity. Potentially useful compounds are next considered for clinical pharmacology.

Clinical trials are conducted to allow safety and efficacy data to be collected for new drugs or devices. These trials can only take place once satisfactory information has been gathered on the quality of the product and its non-clinical safety, and Health Authority/ Ethics Committee approval is granted in the country where the trial is taking place. Depending on the type of product and the stage of its development, investigators enroll healthy volunteers and/or patients into small pilot studies initially, followed by larger scale studies in patients that often compare the new product with the currently prescribed treatment. As positive safety and efficacy data are gathered, the number of patients is typically increased. Clinical trials can vary in size from a single centre in one country to multicentre trials in multiple countries. Due to the sizable cost a full series of clinical trials may incur, the burden of paying for all the necessary people and services is usually borne by the sponsor who may be the pharmaceutical or biotechnology company that developed the agent under study. Since the diversity of roles may exceed resources of the sponsor, often a clinical trial is managed by an outsourced partner such as a contract research organization (CRO).

As mentioned above drug development refers to activities undertaken after a compound is identified as a potential drug in order to establish its suitability as a medication. Objectives of drug development are to determine appropriate Formulation and Dosing, as well as to establish safety. Research in these areas generally includes a combination of *in vitro* studies, *in vivo* studies, and clinical trials. The amount of capital required for late stage development has made it a historical strength of the larger pharmaceutical companies.

Often, large multinational corporations exhibit vertical integration, participating in a broad range of drug discovery and development, manufacturing and quality control, marketing, sales, and distribution. Smaller organizations, on the other hand, often focus on a specific aspect such as discovering drug candidates or developing formulations. Often, collaborative agreements between research organizations and large pharmaceutical companies are formed to explore the potential of new drug substances.

Drug discovery and development is very expensive; of all compounds investigated for use in humans only a small fraction are eventually approved in most nations by government appointed medical institutions or boards, who have to approve new drugs before they can be marketed in those countries. Each year, only about 25 truly novel drugs (new chemical entities) are approved for marketing. This approval comes only after heavy investment in pre-clinical development and clinical trials, as well as a commitment to ongoing safety monitoring. Drugs which fail part-way through this process often incur large costs, while generating no revenue in return. If the cost of these failed drugs is taken into account, the cost of developing a successful new drug (new chemical entity or NCE), has been estimated at about 1 billion USD (not including marketing expenses). A study by the consulting firm Bain and Company reported that the cost for discovering, developing and launching (which factored in marketing and other business expenses) a new drug (along with the prospective drugs that fail) rose over a five year period to nearly $1.7 billion in 2003.

These estimates also take into account the opportunity cost of investing capital many years before revenues are realized (see Time-value of money). Because of the very long time needed for discovery, development, and approval of pharmaceuticals, these costs can accumulate to nearly half the total expense. Some approved drugs, such as those based on re-formulation of an existing active ingredient (also referred to as Line-extensions) are much less expensive to develop. The consumer advocacy group Public Citizen suggests on its web site that the actual cost is under $200 million, about 29% of which is spent on FDA-required clinical trials. For me-too-drugs and for generics, the cost are even less. Calculations and claims in this area are controversial because of the implications for regulation and subsidization of the industry through federally funded research grants.

The Customers

Unlike other product sales, the sale of prescription drug is not based on any choice of the consumer (patient) but rather on that of the physician. So prescription medication sales result from derived demand. Prescription drugs are also known as "directed consumer goods". Actually the physicians/doctors constitutes the major "market" for prescription drugs. Many of the same factors that affect consumer purchase patterns also affect the prescribing habits of the physician. Other recognized factors also influence the physician's decision to prescribe a given medication.

It is important to categorize physicians into general practitioners and specialists. Marketing department of pharmaceutical companies can analyze the number of physicians available in a given specialty so that the pharma company can understand the prescribing habit of physician specialist's, what they prescribe and how much they prescribe, what combination they prescribe, etc. as well as their affinity towards a particular molecule or combination. Identification of physicians by specialty can be helpful to advertisers in determining the size of the physician audience and in finding the relative use of a product by specialists as opposed to general practitioners, though advertisement is not a powerful promotional tool in pharmaceutical marketing.

Pharmaceutical marketers frequently omit physicians over 65 years of age from their direct mail advertising. This is based on the assumption that this group of physicians is less active in practice than their younger counterparts. Age, however, cannot always predict the activity or importance of the physician. Patients, particularly the elderly, tend to continue going to the older physician, with whom they have built up a rapport over the years. Nevertheless, age is a factor in promotional decisions.

The teaching doctor, inspite of his sometimes limited practice is also is one among the target audience of the pharmaceutical company because he influences the future prescribing habits of his students.

In the limited sphere of their use of drugs dentists can be an important source of prescriptions. Among the types of medications administered, prescribed, and dispersed by dentists are narcotic analgesics, non-narcotic analgesics, antibiotics, nasal decongestants, sedatives, tranquilizers, maintenance vitamins, fluoride tablets, fluoride gels, fluoride solutions, fluoride/vitamin combinations, and topical steroids.

Although the area of market opportunity in the field of veterinary medicine is considerably different from that for humans, many of the same drugs are employed, sometimes in the same packages and dosage forms. The field has grown rapidly in recent years, particularly in the small animal field as the nation's pet population has grown in numbers and received increasingly more medical attention.

Various government agencies serve as both direct and indirect marketing for drugs. This segment is also comparatively large.

CONSUMER BEHAVIOUR/PRESCRIBING HABITS

Before understanding about consumer behaviour or prescribing habits and the factors that influence prescribing habits, it is worthy to know what is Prescription and there various functions and its significance in pharmaceutical marketing.

Prescription: By dictionary definition 'prescription' may refer to the directions of administration.

According to The Art of Compounding, prescription is an order written by a physician, dentist, veterinarian, or other licensed practitioner directing the pharmacist to compound and dispense medication for a patient, and usually accompanied by directions for its administration or use.

Functions of the Prescription

Functions of the prescription are divided into: (a) Manifest functions (functions as we perceive them) and (b) Latent functions.

Manifest Functions

1. Means of communication
2. Legal document
3. Record source
4. Method of therapy
5. Means of medical control of therapy
6. Sample mechanism
7. Means of clinical trial

Latent Functions

1. Visible sign of the physician's power to heal
2. Symbol of the power of modern technology
3. Sign that the patient is really ill
4. Legitimizes the long term illness without cure
5. Concrete expressions that physician s has fulfilled his contract
6. Reasonable excuse for human contact with physicians
7. Satisfactorily terminates the visit
8. Fits the concept of modern man that he can control his own destiny
9. Expression of physician's control
10. Indication of physician's concern
11. Medium of communication between physician and patient

12. Forestalls lengthy discussions
13. Source of satisfaction to the physicians
14. Identifies the clinical situation as legitimately medical
15. Legitimizes sick role status
16. Symbol of patient control
17. Means of patient goal attainment.
18. Symbol of patient stability
19. Evidence of physician as an activist
20. Evidence of pharmacist activity
21. Research source of utilization and treatment
22. Medium of exchange
23. Sampling medium
24. Method of clinical trial
25. Method of differentiating legal drug status.

The sale of prescription drug is not based on any choice of the consumer (patient) but rather on that of the physician. Actually the physicians/doctors and all other individuals mentioned above constitutes the major "market" for prescription drugs. Many of the same factors that affect consumer purchase patterns also affect the prescribing habits of the physician. Here we considered the prescriber as the consumer and we depict his behaviour as consumer behaviour or prescribing habit.

Several studies has proved without doubt that physicians goes through a decision making process while prescribing drugs which eventually become their prescribing habit or prescribing behaviour.

Consumer decision making is often classified as rational and emotional. A rational buyer evaluates all alternatives completely, matches his needs with the respective abilities of the products available to fulfill these needs and, theoretically at least, makes his purchase with clear goals in mind. The emotional buyer, on the other hand, may be swayed by product attributes (or the advertising) having nothing to do with the actual need-satisfying properties of the product. It is understood from extensive studies that the basic motivation behind a physician's choice of drug therapy is rational. He would be expected to select the product that would do the most good with the least possible side effects, and perhaps the lowest cost. In most cases of drug selection, however, physicians try to make a rational decision under conditions of uncertainty. Sometimes the customer decision making is based on the combination of rational and emotional motives. This can be true with a physicians prescribing behaviour too. A physician for example may use the most rational therapeutic approach when choosing the proper chemical entity for treating a given condition and then may use completely emotional criteria for the choice of the brand of that drug to employ.

As per scientific studies conducted physician's prescribing a drug for a particular case was a function of: (a) Expectation of the physician that a beneficial effect on the patient's condition would occur if the drug were prescribed, (b) the amount of beneficial effect to be gained by the patient, (c) the expectancy of side effects of the drug, and (d) the magnitude of these side effects.

According to Hemminki the major influences on prescribing are research and the pressures from pharmaceutical companies. Accordingly research and pharmaceutical companies are closely dependent on each other. They may affect the doctors through education, scientific journals and advertising. Doctor's personal characteristics, his working conditions and therapeutic possibilities available as well as patient's personal characteristics, his demands and expectations influences a doctor's drug prescribing habits in a big way. Apart from these factors, control and regulations from health authorities, influences from doctor's professional colleagues, demands and expectations of pressure groups and society at large also has a role to play in a physician's prescribing habit.

Another scientific study conducted among general practitioners using statistical tools concluded that "high curing effect" was uniformly the most important consideration in the selection of a drug to treat hypothetical cases of adult diabetes and pneumonia. "Low side effects" were found to be second in importance in selecting an antidiabetic medication, while "low cost" was found to be more important in selecting an antibiotic. Based on this study, the researcher proposed that physicians select drugs through a habitual or non-habitual choice. Most of the drug choices a physician makes are habitual in nature. When a physician adopt a new drug, he may go through a habitual process (which happens in his mind) which includes components like: (a) Decision criteria, (b) Procedure for gauging the expectations with the decision criteria, (c) Disposition of the drugs and (d) Doctor's knowledge of the drugs. These components or factors help the doctor to take the appropriate drug decision and the outcome of the treatment depends on this.

RR Miller, in his study about adoption of new drugs by doctors summarizes the adoption process under three major subdivisions: (1) Antecedents–factors present in the situation prior to the introduction of new drug, (2) the process and (3) the results.

Antecedents Fall into Two Major Categories

A. Doctor's identity which includes:
   1. Personal characteristics of the doctor like age, experience, orientation and attitude, etc.
   2. Practice characteristics like type of practice, size of practice, patient's income, level of use of class of drugs, etc.
   3. Communication behaviour like detail men, colleagues, cosmopolite sources of information, impersonal sources of information, etc.

B. Doctor's prescriptions of the situation which is influenced by:
   1. Organizational influence,
   2. Cultural and social variables
   3. Patient variables, etc.

C. The drug adoption process through which an individual physician passes from his first hearing of a new drug to his adoption of it. The process can be viewed as consisting of five stages:
   1. Awareness
   2. Interest
   3. Evaluation
   4. Trial
   5. Adoption or rejection

   In the awareness stage the doctor reads or hears about a new drug but has incomplete information about it. In this stage awareness is created in the doctor or he is influenced by information sources like detail man, journal advertising, journal articles, direct mail advertising, samples, meetings, etc.

   He may become interested in the drug and actively seek information in the interest stage.

In this stage sources of information are detail man, journal advertising, journal articles, colleagues, physicians' desk Reference, etc.

In the evaluation stage the physicians mentally applies the new drug to his situation and decides whether or not to try it. In the evaluation stage he gathers information from colleagues, journal articles and through meetings.

In the trial stage the new drug is prescribed on a trial basis to determine its value. Information sources are physicians' desk Reference, journal advertising, house organs, direct mail advertising and samples.

In the final stage which is the adoption stage the physicians begins to use the new drug regularly for all new and perhaps older patients. If the drug does not live up to the standards set it may be rejected also. Other natural outcome of the adoption stages can be continued adoption, later adoption, discontinuance or continued non-adoption.

In the adoption process stage attributes of the new drug like cost, social cost, social reward, and consistency of response, complexity, communicability, pharmaceutical attraction, relative advantage and reputation of the manufacturer are considered by the doctor.

According to the researcher negative factors influencing physician's prescribing are risk and the high continuing cost of therapy.

There are some factors that influence the prescribing of established drugs. They are initial cost of the drug, continuing cost of the drug, social reward, time savings, consistency of therapeutic response, clarity of results, pharmaceutical attractiveness, length of drug name, the name and reputation of manufacturer, etc.

D.B Worthern in his study concludes that six variables influence physician's prescribing habits. They are:

1. Patients
2. Pharmacists
3. Journals
4. Advertising
5. Representatives from pharmaceutical companies

6. Colleagues. The magnitude of influence exerted by each of the variables varied from weak to strong according to the researcher.

A findings of a study conducted by Food and Drug Administration (FDA) in US were the following:

1. Estimated readership among physicians for national journals is highest for specialty journals (the Journal of the American Medical Association has the highest overall readership);
2. The most widely used and most often consulted source of drug information is the Physicians' Desk Reference;
3. Package inserts are the most used source of information among drug company materials,
4. Peer colleagues followed by consultants are the most often used sources among personal contacts,
5. Textbooks are used less frequently for drug information, and
6. Sources of drug information strong in believability, currency, and provision of the best clinical guidance are national journal articles, meetings, and courses.

A study about sources of drug information conducted on dentists revealed that published or editorial matter ranked first among dentists surveyed, and detail men and advertisements in dental publications ranked second. The former received a higher percentage of first-place rankings and the latter received more third-place rankings.

Role of Patient

a. In spite of the importance of the doctors in the choice of prescription medications, patient (ultimate consumer) choice still demands thorough consideration. Usually a person has a choice in what he does about his health. He can choose to have a checkup or not to have a checkup. The patient has the freedom to choose his physicians, his pharmacist and ultimately although his influence may be indirect determines the components of total health care. Apart from the doctor who takes various decisions on the treatment, the patient also is involved in decision making activity because illness is an altered state of well-being about which an individual has to take series of decisions. As per

Andrew Twaddle the major decision making areas for a patient (individual) are as follows:

b. That some change from normal health has occurred (some symptoms have shown up or routine checkups would have found out something abnormal).

c. That the change is significant (the patient considers that the change is significant is usually based on various factors).

d. That help is needed (even if the symptom is significant not all the patients will decide to take help. Some may resort to self medication. Factors like perceived morbidity, anxiety, age, sex, race, financial conditions, etc. has a role to play in deciding whether help is needed or not).

e. That a particular type of help is preferable (choice of type of help will be a function of social, cultural, economic, educational, emotional, geographic and legal factors).

f. That a particular treatment agent or setting is appropriate (Many factors plays a role while deciding on a particular doctor/ hospital/pharmacist. Some of the factors are: Convenient location (close to home, close to work, close to shopping, close to doctor in case of selecting pharmacy). Parking space available, less waiting time, professional and convenient service, like the person, etc.

In case of pharmacy selection: (Professional service, price better than other pharmacies, personal attention, a pharmacist who knows your physician, a ready source of drug information, advertised drug price, quality and merchandise assortments, etc.) By and large the patients expect and indeed want professional attention and services.

g. That certain types and degrees of cooperation with the treatment agent are appropriate. Patient's cooperation is very important for successful therapy. The major factors affecting patient cooperation are:

Demographic	: Age and income of patient
Structural	: Cost and duration.
Patient attitudes	: Towards medical contact experience
Interaction	: With physician
Enabling	: Prior experience, source of advice

As cost of drug is a major factor affecting patient cooperation, we may look into the various cost factors.

Cost for Patient

Cost for patient includes

1. Cost of prescription
2. Cost of drug per day
3. Cost for partially versus entirely filing the prescription
4. Cost of total treatment
5. Proportion of total treatment cost
6. Its position in cost sequence
7. Perceived cost
8. Expected cost
9. Past cost experiences
10. Importance of the cost, based on the ability to pay
11. Opportunity cost (what is given up to purchase the drug)
12. Convenience or inconvenience of dosage form used in improving compliance
13. Psychic or symbolic cost
14. Cost of alternatives, including noncompliance
15. Cost of competing products, their generic equivalence or nonequivalence and their therapeutic effectiveness
16. Non-economic costs—like the time the patient spends to get a prescription filled, psycho logic costs in admitting that one is ill enough to need a prescription, etc.

These cost factors may affect the patient's purchasing or not purchasing of drugs. High cost of drugs would deter patient cooperation in one or more of the following ways:

1. Fail to fill prescription.
2. Fail to refill medication.
3. Fail to take consume drugs as frequently as prescribed.
4. Discontinuing medication prematurely to preserve some drugs for a future episode of illness.

On the contrary patients who pay high price for the medicine may use the drug more meticulously and responsibly, as he has paid more. All these factors call for the doctors' consideration individually or in combination. Some of these factors that may inhibit the patient from getting the prescription filled initially may actually promote cooperation once that step is taken.

Pharmaceutical Product

A product is anything that can be offered to a market for attention, acquisition , use or consumption and might satisfy a want or need. Product refer to tangible and intangible goods like physical objects, services, events, persons, places, organizations, ideas or combinations of these. In the total marketing offering, product is a key element. Marketing mix planning starts with formulating an offer that brings value to target customers, and satisfies their specific needs.

Levels of Product

- Core benefit
- Basic product
- Expected product
- Augmented product
- Potential product.

Products have five levels, which are known as 'consumer value hierarchy', with each level adding more customer value. The most basic level is the core product or core benefit. This is what the customer is actually buying. At the second level the core benefit is turned into a basic product. This will have features, designs, a quality level, a brand name and packaging. At the third level, it becomes an expected product, a set of attributes and conditions normally expected by consumers when they buy the product. At the forth level, it becomes an augmented product by offering additional consumer services and benefits that exceed customer expectations. Finally it becomes the potential product, containing all the possible augmentations and transformations that it might undergo in the future.

Products can be classified into two classes on the type of consumers who use them:

1. Consumer products
2. Industrial products

Consumer products are products and services bought by final consumers for personal consumption. Industrial products are purchased for further production, processing or for use in conducting a business.

Pharmaceutical products fall under consumer products as they are brought by final consumers or patients for their consumption or for the consumption of their family members. Pharmaceutical products are more commonly known as medicines or drugs and are a fundamental component of both modern and traditional medicine. It is essential that such products are safe, effective, and of good quality, and are prescribed and used rationally.

Pharmaceutical products in India can be broadly divided into:

1. Allopathic
2. Ayuervedic
3. Unani
4. Sidda
5. Homeopathy
6. Naturopathy and Yoga

Pharmaceutical products can be further divided into:

1. Prescription drugs
2. Non-prescription drugs

Prescription's Drugs

Prescription drugs are drugs that are not locally available without a physician's prescription. The major prescription drugs are:

1. Anti-convulsant drugs
2. Anti-angina drugs
3. Anti-fungal drugs
4. Anti-itch drugs
5. Anti-viral drugs
6. Anti-diabetic drugs
7. Anti-asthmatic drugs
8. Anti-hypertensive drugs
9. Antibiotics
10. Anti-migraine drugs
11. Anti-rheumatic drugs
12. Anti-protozoal drugs

13. Tricyclic anti-depressants
14. Anti-arrhythmic drugs
15. Anti-nausea drugs
16. Anti-Parkinson drugs
17. Anti-psychotic drugs
18. Muscle relaxants
19. Digitalis drugs
20. Anti-gastroesophageal reflux drugs
21. Anti-retroviral drugs
22. Anti-tuberculosis drugs
23. Anti-ulcer drugs
24. Anti-hemorrhoid drugs
25. Anti-spasmodic drugs
26. Anti-malarial drugs
27. Non-steroidal anti-inflammatory drugs: Some can be bought over the counter; others are available only with a prescription from a physician or dentist.
28. Immuno-suppressant drugs
29. Anti-insomnia drugs
30. Anti-helminthic drugs
31. Central nervous system stimulants
32. Decongestants: Some decongestant products require a physician's prescription but there are also many non-prescription (over-the-counter) products.
33. Anti-coagulant Drugs
34. Bone disorder drugs
35. Infertility drugs
36. Topical antibiotics: Some topical antibiotics are available with a prescription only.
37. Diuretics
38. Vasodilators: In the forms used for treating high blood pressure (tablets or injections), these drugs are available only with a physician's prescription.
39. Blood-viscosity reducing drugs
40. Beta-blockers
41. Corticosteroids
42. Benzodiazepines

43. Cephalosporins
44. Expectorants: Some products that contain are available only with a physician's prescription
45. Sulfonamides
46. Calcium channel blockers
47. Gout drugs
48. Anti-histamines: Some anti-histamine products are available only with a physician's prescription.
49. Penicillins
50. Barbiturates
51. Laxatives
52. ACE inhibitors
53. Anti-anxiety drugs
54. Urinary anti-infectives
55. MAO inhibitors
56. Opioid analgesics
57. Bronchodilators
58. Ophthalmic antibiotics
59. Smoking cessation drugs: Some products are available only with a prescription.
60. Protease inhibitor
61. Anti-depressant drugs
62. Alpha1 adrenergic blockers
63. Tetracyclines.

Non-prescription Drugs

These are medicines, which can be bought at a pharmacy without the prescription of a doctor, at the pharmacist's advice.

1. Anti-hemorrhoid drugs
2. Topical antibiotics: Some topical antibiotics are available without a prescription
3. Cough-suppressants
4. Anti-acne drugs
5. Non-steroidal anti-inflammatory drugs: Some can be bought over the counter; others are available only with a prescription from a physician or dentist.
6. Antiseptics

7. Analgesics
8. Decongestants: Some decongestant products require a physician's prescription but there are also many non-prescription (over-the-counter) products.
9. Aspirin
10. Vasodilators: Some vasodilators such as Minoxidil are sold without prescription.
11. Antacids
12. Expectorants: Many expectorants are available without a physician's prescription.
13. Anti-fungal drugs
14. Anti-histamines: Some can be bought without prescription.
15. Anti-gas agents
16. Smoking cessation drugs: Many drugs can be bought over the counter, without prescription.

Pharmaceutical products are segmented on the basis of their therapeutic usage. The major therapeutic groups are:

1. Respiratory
2. Cholesterol and triglyceride reducers
3. Anti-ulcerents
4. Anti-depressants
5. Anti-psychotics
6. Anti-epileptics
7. Anti-rheumatic
8. Anti-diabetic
9. Cephalosporin's and combinations
10. Erythropoietin's
11. Calcium antagonists.

Pharmaceutical Product Decisions

Three types of product decisions are normally involved in pharmaceutical marketing. They are:

1. Individual product decisions
2. Product line decisions
3. Product mix decisions.

Individual Product Decisions Involved

a. Product attributes
b. Branding
c. Packaging
d. Labeling.

Product attributes: The benefits offered by a product are delivered by product attributes such as quality, feature, design, etc. product quality is the ability of a product to perform its promised functions. Product features are a competitive tool used to differentiate the company's product in the market.

Branding: It is an important tool for pharmaceutical marketers to create separate identity for a company's product. A brand is a name, term, sign, symbol, or design or a combination of these that identifies the maker or seller of a product. Branding adds value to a product and consumers view a brand as an important part of a product the marketers or sellers have various advantages in branding. The brand name becomes the basis of which a whole story can be built about a product's special attributed and qualities. The seller's brand name and trade mark provide legal protection for unique product features that otherwise might be copied by competitors. Branding helps sellers to establish brand image, brand personality, brand equity and brand loyalty for products. Branding also facilitate the marketer to segment markets and practice differential marketing.

Pharmaceutical brands vary in the amount of power and value they have in the market. A powerful brand has high brand equity. Brand equity is positive differential effect that knowing the brand name has on consumer response to the product or service. A measure of brand's equity is the extent to which consumers are willing to pay more for the brand. A brand with strong brand equity is a very valuable asset for any company and it enjoys a high level of consumer brand awareness and loyalty. Since the brand name carries high credibility the company can more easily launch line and brand extensions. So it is important for pharmaceutical marketers to develop there products into sucesssful brands with high brand equity. Major decisions areas in brand strategy decisions in pharmaceutical products are brand name selection, brand sponsorship and brand development.

Pharmaceutical companies use various brand strategies to develop and strengthen their brands. The common brand strategies are:

1. Individual brand strategy wherein each individual product in a single product class is given a separate brand name. Individual branding, also called multibranding, is the marketing strategy of giving each product in a product portfolio its own unique brand name. This is contrasted with family branding in which the products in a product line are given the same brand name. The advantage of individual branding is that each product has a self image and identity that's unique. This facilitates the positioning process. That means that there are less Halo-effects and one can position all products differently without making trade-offs.
2. Family brand strategy wherein a common brand name is given to all related products. Family branding is a marketing strategy that involves selling several related products under one brand name. It is contrasted with individual branding in which each product in a portfolio is given a unique identity and brand name. There are often economies of scale associated with family branding since several products can efficiently be promoted with a single advertisement or campaign. Family branding facilitates new product introductions by providing a 'foot-in-the-door' in potential customers' evoked set. When considering purchasing a new type of product, potential customers tend to evoke in their minds a product with a familiar brand name. Being a part of this evoked set can lead to trial purchase, product acceptance, or other advantages. Family brand strategy is commonly used because a number of drugs have to be used in different dosage forms for different indications and for different age groups. Here the company encashes the image of a highly successful and popular brand name.
3. Corporate brand strategy where in the company name is used for the products, so that the positive and favorable image of the company can be used successfully for selling the company products.
4. Pharmaceutical companies also use multiple brand strategy in which the same product is sold or marketed in two or more brand names so that a bigger market share can be achieved. Glaxo has

achieved 45% of market share in multivitamin-mineral market using this strategy.

A study conducted in USA about Pharmaceutical Brand Leadership: Getting There and Staying on - why do some pharmaceutical brands fail and others succeed? This study identifies exact factors driving some brands such as Celebrex and Lipitor to the front of the pack in their therapeutic classes and what kept these brands at #1. With this knowledge, marketing teams can empower themselves to shape the destiny of a brand knowing what activities and skills truly make a difference in the journey to market leader. They can drive brands—regardless of their clinical differentiation—to the levels of proven winners!

To identify these success factors connected to winning brands, the researcher surveyed 15 companies about marketing activities and capabilities and overall success factors and interviewed 6 executives with titles that include vice-president, directors of marketing, sales manager and product/brand manager to capture their perspectives on what made a brand a hit. The companies selected were Astra Zeneca, Abbott Laboratories, Amgen, Aventis, Baxter Healthcare, Biogen, Bayer, Boehringer-Ingelheim, GlaxoSmithKline, Johnson & Johnson, Pfizer, Roche, TAP, UCB Pharma and Wyeth.

Along with other rankings, executives rank—according to their ance to brand leadership — internal and external factors, such as:

- Expanding marketing resources,
- Launching new indications,
- Garnering favorable reimbursement,
- Modifying treatment guidelines,
- Shifting competitor priorities,
- Loss of thought leader support for a competitor, and
- Expiring patents.

The study finds out from 82% in the benchmark class that currently are leaders in the marketplace what activities, capabilities and resources propelled them ahead of their peers. Such metrics include how internal clinical and marketing capabilities and skills rank in the assessment of what makes a winning brand formula. For example, how important is the collecting and tracking of health outcomes to brand success compared with advocacy management? Executives behind current leading brands reveal their opinions.

When asked about the overall success factor mix elements kept their brands on the top (success factors and mix elements—1. Clinical differentiation, 2. Marketing differentiation and 3. Sales force effectiveness) executives mentioned that a fairly even mix of clinical differentiation (42%) marketing differentiation (36%) and sales force effectiveness (22%) made this possible. There is a slight trend toward clinical differentiation as being the most important factor.

The study reveals that companies realize it is often not enough to spend like your competitor. In fact, you have to outspend the competition, especially in areas such as market research, patient education and journal advertising, to make significant impact on their position in the market.

The study has revealed that fostering competitive intelligence is important to keep a close eye on competitor activities and spending. Companies that want their product to reach #1 in the market must invest in a variety of competitive intelligence initiatives from offensive and defensive positions.

Key activities from an offensive position are Site monitors, science mapping, conference intelligence, war games. Matrix plotting, performance measures, lifecycle profiles and scenario planning.

Key activities under defensive position are database archives, Internet portals, competitive landscapes, trend analysis, search engines, published articles, data dumping and secondary sources.

Generic *vs* Brand Names for Medicines

Generic name: Each medicine (drug) has an approved name called the *generic* name. A group of medicines that have similar actions often have similar sounding generic names. For example, penicillin, ampicillin, amoxicillin and flucloxacillin are in one group of antibiotics.

Brand name: Many medicines also have one or more *brand* names. This is chosen by the company that makes it. Several companies may make the same medicine, each with their own brand name. The name is often chosen to be memorable for advertising, or to be easier to say or spell than some long generic name! For example, paracetamol is a generic name. There are several companies that make this with brand names such as Panadol, Calpol, etc.

The brand name is usually written most clearly on any packaging. However, you will always see the generic name written somewhere on the packet (often in small print). Some medicines only have the generic name on the packet.

The color, size, shape, etc. of brands of the same medicine may vary depending on which company makes it. Do not be alarmed if your regular medicine seems to have changed color or shape. It may be that the pharmacist is getting it from a different company, or the doctor has written the prescription in a generic way rather than using a brand name. However, the medicine will be the same if the generic name is the same as before.

Combination Products

Some products contain a combination of medicines. Combination products have one brand name. However, the individual ingredients will all be listed in small print on the packet. For example, a popular painkiller has a brand name of Solpadine. This contains three generic medicines— Paracetamol, codeine, and caffeine.

Generic Prescribing

Doctors are encouraged to prescribe by using the generic name. This is because: The generic name is the one doctors are trained to use. There are sometimes many brand names for one medicine. Possible confusion or mistakes are reduced if all doctors use the same names when talking about and prescribing medicines.

Generic medicines are often cheaper for the NHS. Even for medicines that you can buy, such as paracetamol, there is often a big price difference between brands.

Some Leading Pharmaceutical Brands

Pfizer	-	Lipitor, Norvasc, Zoloft
Wyeth	-	Effexor, Protonix, Prevnar
GlaxoSmithKline	-	Seretide, Avandia, Seroxat
Merck	-	Zocor, Fosamax, Cozaar
Eli Lilly	-	Zyprexa
Bayer	-	Cipro

Packaging: Packaging involves the activities of designing and producing the container or wrapper of a product. The package should be capable of communicating quality, economy, prestige, relief, etc. Colour, design, shape, size, brand name , materials, labels and typography are the components of packaging communication process. Each of these components must interact harmoniously and synchronize to evoke the desired responses in the consumer.

Functions of Packaging (Packaging as a Marketing Tool)

- It contains and protect the product
- Package is a silent salesman
- It attracts attention, describes the product
- Creates customer confidence
- Creates instant product and brand recognition
- Creates competitive advantage to company.
- It communicates various features like quantity or weight of contents, ingredients used, brand name, manufacturers or marketers identity, usage pattern occasion, dosage, etc. price, instructions to use and other messages.

Labelling: Product, brand and price information printed on the package is labelling. It can vary from simple tags attached to products to complex graphics that are part of the package.

- Label identifies the product or brand
- Describes manufacturer's name, place of manufacture, date, content using instructions, safety precaution, etc.
- Label promotes the product.

In pharmaceutical products packaging has a limited role to play, i.e. a functional role because pharmaceutical products in general and ethical drugs in particular are not purchased by the patient on impulse, but is prescribed by a physician. As the pharmaceutical industry is regulated by the government, packaging has to be done according to the guidelines given by Food and Drug Administration. Safety and stability are the most important factors considered in packaging. FDA gives clear guideline about all important aspects to be considered while designing pharmaceutical product packages. FDA also prescribes the colours to be used for printing the brand name and the company logo. Cost effective packaging is important in pharmaceutical products because pharmaceutical companies are not allowed to exceed the limit of input cost fixed by the government.

Product Life Cycle

With a lot of effort going into new product development, firms have the benefit of introducing new products. Care should be taken in managing the new introduction to ensure profits and volume business. Later on during the growth, maturity and decline stages of the PLC proper management is required.

A product has a life cycle and it asserts four things:

1. Products have limited life.
2. Product sales pass through distinct stages, each posing different challenges, opportunities, and problems to the seller.
3. Profits rise and fall at different stages of the product life cycle.
4. Products require different marketing, financial, manufacturing, purchasing and human resource strategies in each life cycle stage.

The product life cycle and marketing activities of the firm are thoroughly interrelated. Each stage of the life cycle of a particular type of product is characterized by different market conditions and marketing activities. On the other hand, the marketing activities of the firm affect the life cycle. The pharmaceutical market is also characterized by periodic replacement of top-selling products by new entries. New product which is either a new chemical entity or a modification of an existing product is launched in the market, as pharmaceutical companies are aggressively involved in research and development. Because of their own active research and development programmes and, more importantly, because of similar programmes of competing companies, most firms find that their new products experience some variation of a basic life cycle. Variations on this cycle occur primarily in the length of the five phases and in the magnitude of the sales volume. There seems to be little doubt that the concept of product life cycle can be applied to pharmaceuticals as well. The mandate of this cycle for research development is clear. New drugs are necessary for survival. No firm can afford the luxury of resting on its laurels following the successful development and introduction of a new product. History has proven that competing firms will quickly make such rest an uneasy one.

Some authors have opined that a medicine's life cycle begins with an initial research activity, continues with production and sales under patent to the final stage of competition with generic products.

Introduction Stage

In the introduction stage a new class of medicine is presented to the physician for the first time. There can be two types of new products. One is a medicine that does something old in a new way, and the second one is that does something that was not possible before. Increase in sales is generally slow in this stage as the physician habits must be broken, at least to the extent of trying the new product. The process may be fast if the medical profession has been awaiting this type of development for a long time. The market for the product during this phase will be small. It comprises of physicians who are the first to try new drugs, and who are opinion leaders and quite influential with their colleagues. If the product is as effective and safe to fulfill there needs, the introduction will be comparatively fast as this will lead to word of mouth publicity within doctor's community. The ease of introduction of a new product class can be expected to be affected by the relative success of any previous efforts in this product class.

In the introductory stage direct competition may not be a problem although, if the product merely does a job in a new or better way, there may be difficulty in convincing the physician of the value of a change. Production cost, marketing costs, and prices are traditionally high during the introduction stage. Unless the product can be produced efficiently using existing equipment and in the face of unpredictable sales, the economics of mass production will be hard to realize. If the new product represents a sufficiently radical departure from traditional therapy, it may conceivably be necessary to familiarize the physician, with the new concept. The distribution portion of marketing costs will also be higher than normal, with the special problems of initial stocking of pharmacies and hospitals.

Usually in the introduction stage the price of the medicine will be the highest. This reflects both the lack of direct competition and the uncertain sales future. Even at this highest price, in the face of high production and marketing costs and with the buildup of past research and development costs, management may plan on operating at a loss on the product during the introductory stage.

In short the introductory phase is a phase of market development. The duration of the introductory stage depends on the degree of newness of the medicine, its complexity, and its ability to cater to the needs of the target customers, the physicians.

Growth Stage

Growth stage of the medicine is characterized by its widespread acceptance among the target audience. If the product successfully survives the introduction stage, it can be expected that many more physicians will start prescribing the new medicine. As the demand for the medicine increases in the growth phase, the market also expands as the number of competitors goes up during this stage. Competitors may introduce either modifications of the original product or completely different products for the same purpose. By this time production methods will have been established, with a frequent lowering of costs. During this stage prices may go down due to increased sales and increased competition. Both these factors may force the pharmaceutical company to lower the price of the medicine which is introduced successfully. During this stage the manufacturer devotes the promotional activities to stimulate selective demand. Promotional activities will be aimed at popularizing the advantages of the new brand in comparison with those of the competitors. Detailing stories will contain comparison between company's product and competitor's products.

Maturity Stage

Competition reaches its peak during the maturity stage. Most of the pharma companies who anticipates grabbing reasonable market share would have already introduced their brand, by this time. All potential customers probably would have accepted the brand by the time it reaches maturity stage. The total sales which have been rising through the early stages, continue to increase, but at a decreasing rate. Efforts to sell to large volume buyers like hospitals and government agencies also becomes heated during this stage, which will result in increased price competition. As far as promotion is concerned the emphasis from medical representatives who details the product changes to journal advertising and direct mail during this stage.

Saturation Stage

The point at which the drug has been tried and used for all remotely feasible indications and has found its place in the therapeutic resources of the physician indicates the saturation point. New sales from this point on are strictly a function of population and incidence of disease. The physician community may also realize and doubt the efficiency of the product. During this phase all the product variations like tablets, capsules, liquid , dermatologic form, a long-acting form, or a combination may appear. In the saturation stage the number of competitors of any importance stabilizes. Indeed, because of the effectiveness of earlier selective demand stimulation, it would probably be difficult for any new firm to penetrate the market at all. The promotional efforts may now target different market segments by using special messages to separate physician specialties.

Decline

Decline of a product class is usually related to the effectiveness of the product as compared to other means of therapy. The decline will be rapid if the decline is caused by a new product development. Physicians who are slow to change only may continue to prescribe the product. Promotion during this stage may again be aimed at stimulation of primary demand. The effort may be half-hearted, and may be aimed at only a core of physician-users. Some firms may now drop from the competition, leaving a potential marketing opportunity for those remaining. The profits may be slim, however, with many of the economies gone.

The length of life cycle for pharmaceutical products is neither predictable nor uniform. When some product types come and go so quickly others remain in vogue for years. There is no real uniformity in the respective length of the stages. Decline may be rapid or quite slow.

It is important for pharmaceutical companies to extend a product life cycle so to ensure better profits and maximize return on investments. This can be done by developing new delivery systems and new indications, by developing consumer pull, reinventing product portfolios and by switching to OTC or competing in the generic market, by entering new markets , by expanding existing market coverage, modifying products, introducing different pack sizes, introducing new flavors, etc.

Product Life Cycle Management (PLM)

Product Life Cycle Management is widely used by progressive pharmaceutical companies in India and abroad to manage their products. Product life cycle management is the succession of strategies used by management as a product goes through its product life cycle. The conditions in which a product is sold changes over time and must be managed as it moves through its succession of stages. PLM has more to do with managing descriptions and properties of a product through its development and useful life, mainly from a business/engineering point of view.

Product Management (Product Director/Product Manager)

Most pharmaceutical companies have appointed product directors (usually in western pharmaceutical companies) or product managers (usually in Indian pharmaceutical companies) who are concerned with developing market plans for existing products and also new product development.

The principal functional responsibilities of the product director are the following:

- Develop business and marketing strategies and plans.
- Manage strategies and plans about pricing, distribution, labelling, trademarking, and packaging associated with assigned products.
- Establish and achieve all quantifiable product/project/personnel objectives.
- Develop unit and dollar sales projections to ensure appropriate planning to meet the anticipated needs of the marketplace and achievement of profit plans.
- Develop appropriate new dosage forms strategy and plans for assigned products to maximize opportunities.
- Conduct team meetings, foster communications among team members and departments, and issue appropriate and timely minutes.
- Work with sales management to achieve national and regional sales strategies and plans.
- Direct selected projects that will impact across product lines and influence future business policies of the firm.
- Ensure, through leadership and direction, that the planning, developing, implementation, and monitoring of marketing programmes conform with and fully support the product plan.

- Initiate and maintain appropriate linkage between the product and project teams and other functional resources, such as distribution, drug regulatory affairs, finance, law, materials management, product development, packaging development, production, manufacturing, facilities planning, research, public relations, public policy, business development, and strategic planning.
- Communicate and actively participate with research and project management to ensure that product research and development plans are implemented that fulfills agreed-to strategies for assigned products and therapeutic areas.
- Coordinate to achieve mutually satisfactory resolution of any actual or potential conflicts identified between assigned product marketing strategies or programmes and existing local, state, or federal laws and regulations.
- Monitor social, political, economic, regulatory, and legal trends affecting the pharmaceutical industry and assigned markets and react with recommendations.
- Consult with and engage outside support, consultants, and agencies to ensure the continuous generation of new, innovative and creative ideas for product and project objectives.
- Establish budgets, budget mix and monitor expenditure by specific media and target audiences for products or projects.
- Anticipate and apprise management of changes in the market place and initiate modifications to the marketing plan based on evolving market dynamics.
- Exercise final team approval on promotional copy and field communications related to assigned products.
- Assume responsibility in concert with appropriate department heads to assist team members in the informal training process relative to team interactions and activities.
- Participate and interact with broad chartered committees, such as FDA production committee, product coordinating committee, project teams, and product management review committee.
- Coordinate the response to FDA relative to assigned marketed products with drug regulatory affairs and others.
- Input into project management to maximize potential marketing opportunities prior to issuance of the transfer document.
- Review and comment on selling emphasis programmes.

- Recommend appropriate allocation of sales efforts for the pharmaceutical line to the sales department and marketing board for the current planning period.
- Launch new products.

The role of product managers in Indian scenario is very limited as compared to their western counterparts. There major responsibilities are:

1. Helping the field staff by preparing detailing stories for the products assigned to them. Assisting and guiding he field force in terms of retail audit, promotional strategies, supply of promotional materials, detailing stories, etc.
2. Directing the field staff on sampling, i.e. what products to be sampled, how much to be sampled, to which doctors to be sampled and how much to be sampled to different profile of doctors.
3. Monitoring own product movement and competitor's product movement in the market.
4. Monitoring and analyzing product wise and region wise product demand and sales, and reporting to higher ups.

THE PHARMACEUTICAL PLACE

Distribution decisions are critical in nature as they affect the viability of the firm and the product. These decisions affect the market share of the firm and hence great care has to be taken in selecting distribution alternatives. Inspite of all your product superiority and attributes if it is not made available in the right place in the right time and in the right quantity the product will not be able to perform in the market. Reaching out to the market, therefore, holds the key to the competitive advantage of firms. Reaching out to the market involves planning and strateging at two levels–distribution structure and logistics. The distribution structure refers to the channel design and structure, and management of channels. Logistics refers to the physical aspect of distribution.

Distribution Channels

- Manufacturer
- The wholesaler

- The pharmacist
- Consumer.

Manufacturer

Pharmaceutical companies are concerned in manufacturing or processing of drugs into pharmaceutical preparations for human or veterinary use. As the pharmaceutical preparations industry accounts for over 90% of the total medicines consumed (especially in India) Ayurvedic drugs which consists of herbal and botanical drugs does not come under the purview of this topic for the time being.

Pharmaceutical companies or the pharmaceutical manufacturers which is the first in the distribution channel should be characterized by financial strength, good reputation and progressive and structured business policies. One of the important decisions that firms have to take is regarding the number of channel levels to serve a given market as well as the length and width of distribution channel. The length of the channel is often determined by factors like size of the market, order size lot, service requirements, product variety, etc.

Distribution decisions of pharmaceutical companies are not taken in void. Factors like market characteristics, company characteristics, product characteristics, middleman characteristics, intensity of competition and environmental characteristics have to be taken into serious consideration by pharmaceutical manufacturers before deciding distribution patterns, channel objectives and constraints. Pharmaceutical companies have the choice of selecting appropriate channel members. Some companies prefer to sell their products through Super stockiest – stockiest – retailer channel. Usually new market entrants use this method. Some companies appoints C&F agents instead of Super stockiest. The channel structure will be C&F agent – stockiest – retailer. Some companies opt for Company own depot instead of C&F agents. The structure is Company own depot–stockiest–retailer. Large companies like Glaxo and Sandoz however follows a combination of different structures. They have company own deport as well as C&F system depending on various market conditions and other factors.

Wholesaler

Wholesalers who are step 2 in the pharmaceutical distribution channel purchases goods from the drug manufacture sells them to other wholesalers, retailers, pharmacies, medical shops, hospitals, nursing homes and dispensing doctors. Wholesalers can be classified into.

1. Super stockiest
2. Stockiest
3. Sub-stockiest
4. Clearing and forwarding agents (C&F agents)

Super stockiest are appointed by manufacturers to look after the entire distribution function of their products. Usually super stockiest is appointed to handle distribution of a complete state or part of a state. Size of the geographical territory (state), volume of business, planned degree of market penetration, etc. are some of the considerations to appoint super stockiest. A super stockiest sells the drugs of the of the company to stockinet's appointed by the company, as well as to hospitals, nursing homes and dispensing doctors.

1. ***The functions of super stockiest includes:***
   i. Maintaining adequate stocks of the entire range of products manufactured/marketed by the company.
   ii. Reselling these products to stockiest as well as to hospitals, nursing homes and dispensing doctors.
   iii. Providing territoty wise sales data (territory covered by super stockiest), stock position, stockiest wise outstanding payment data to the company periodically (month wise, quarterly wise) etc.
   iv. Collection and replacement of returned goods.
2. ***Stockist:*** Stockiest are appointed by pharmaceutical companies to supply their pharma products to retailers (chemists and druggists, etc.) hospitals, nursing homes and dispensing doctors. Stockists who are 3rd in the distribution channel purchases company goods on from a super stockist and not a directly form the company and caters to smaller territory as compared to super stockist. Depending on situation stockiest may or may not supply products to sub-stockiest. The functions of stockiest are similar

to super stockiest. Almost all data generated by the super stockiest are also generated by stockiest and given to the company directly or when the medical representative visits them. The most important function of the stockiest is market penetration. As they operate in small geographical territories they can understand the pulse of the market better than super stockiest. Stockiest maintain closer interaction with chemists and druggists, so are very close to market reactions.

3. ***Sub-stockists***: For better market penetration and reach stockiest may appoint sub- stockists. Sub-stockists function in a relatively smaller geographical are and their functions are similar to stockiest.
4. ***Carry and Forward (C&F) agents:*** Unlike super stockiest C&F agent does not purchase goods from the company and it virtually operates like a company distributor office or depot. Carry and Forward agent manages the distribution function on behalf of the pharma company for a mutually agreed commission. The commission payable to the C&F agent varies from company to company and usually depends upon the sales turnover of the company. The commission can be a fixed amount every month irrespective of sales volume. Even this fixed amount is usually based on the volume of present as well as projected sales. Usually the commission varies from 1.5 to 3%. Most of the pharmaceutical companies takes a security deposit equivalent to one month sales from C&F agents, in the form of a bank guarantee.

Most of the functions performed by C&F agents and superstockist are similar in nature except for few. Carry and Forward agent have additional functions like:

1. Dispatching companies promotional materials like sample and gifts to the field force.
2. Monitoring documentation procedure and submission of sales tax in time.

Retailer (Chemists or Druggists)

The next step in the pharmaceutical distribution channel is the retailer commonly known as chemist or druggists. He can be a hospital pharmacist also. The chemist holds stock of important and essential medicine as well provides supplementary information required by patients regarding price, dosage, side effects, etc. Since pharmaceutical products are concerned with the health of the people it is essential that the persons who dispense the drugs on the prescriptions of doctors possess adequate technical knowledge only then, can they interact and communicate with consumers regarding maters related to the dosage side effects drug interactions, etc. Therefore in India it is mandatory that retail chemist or druggist should be qualified and licensed to sell pharmaceutical preparations and the minimum qualification for a registered pharmacist, who can dispense medicines on the prescription of a medical practitioner, is a Diploma in Pharmacy. The selling of prescription pharmaceuticals to the public is thus restricted to the comparatively small numbers of pharmacists and pharmacies in the country rather than to the substantially larger number of retailers and retail outlets that would normally be the case for a consumer product.

In pharmaceutical distribution channel the role played by chemists or druggists are vital as compared to all other pharmaceutical distribution channel members. This is because it is the chemist who dispenses the prescription of a medical practitioner and sell medicines to a patient. Product availability at the retail counter is most crucial. If a prescription is returned or dishonored for want of stocks the doctor usually changes that prescription and suggests an alternative. Many a times the chemist himself may dispense an alternative brand in case of dishonor of prescription. To make a doctor prescribe a brand is twice as difficult as getting his prescription in the first place. Pharmaceutical company's field staff therefore has to ensure that their product is available with the chemist before they detail their product to the doctor. They have to develop good rapport with the chemist so to ensure success in sales. Apart from this the chemist can help the company in pushing the sales of the company's OTC formulations and also prescriptions drugs with OTC profile.

Chemists are very good source or the only source of prescription data. Prescription audit data is a technique used by companies' measures the outflow of prescription drugs from the pharmacy into the hands of the consumer. In many ways, it may be logically argued that prescription audit data are the most sensitive indicators of prescription product performance in the marketplace. Chemists are also very important source of information regarding the prescribing behaviour of the doctors around him and the movement of products of various competitors. The prescription is not an expression of opinion, attitude, or speculation on the part of the prescriber but is a matter of record. As prescribers collectively change their minds about individual drugs or areas of therapy these changes are, in essence, automatically recorded in the prescription files of pharmacies. Prescriptions, further, are indicators of what is presently occurring in terms of demand. Purchase data, for example, may record a pharmacy's purchase of antibiotics in the month of August in anticipation of the antibiotic "season." That purchase record, however, does not signify current physician demand for antibiotics. Prescription data are also viewed by most pharmaceutical marketers as the best indicators of the results of marketing or promotional efforts to create new business. If one looks at purchase data for an antihypertensive product it is impossible to sort-out that portion of dollars representative of new business as opposed to that portion reflective of patients who are already using the product. New prescription volume for the same product, however, is a reasonably good indicator of the trend in generating new patient business for the product. Successful medical representatives realize the importance of the chemist and spend good amount of time with him to gather valuable information. Lot of quality information can be gathered from bill books, stock register and prescriptions brought by patients.

Institutional Market

The pharmaceutical institutional market includes purchases made by

- Director general of suppliers and disposals
- Medical stores depots
- Railway hospitals
- Employees state Insurance Corporation
- Armed Forces Medical Stores Depots
- Central Government Health Scheme
- Hospitals in public sector undertakings
- Hospitals attached to medical colleges
- Government hospitals

- Primary health centers
- Private hospitals

The pharmaceutical manufacturer either sells his products directly to institutions or through middlemen. Due to delay in payments from institution most of the pharmaceutical companies in India appoint a special hospital distributor to sell their products to institutions.

Supply Chain Management and Logistics

Physical distribution has now been expanded into the broader concept of supply chain management. Supply chain management starts before physical distribution; it involves procuring the right inputs (raw materials, components and capital equipment), converting them efficiently into finished products and dispatching them to the final destinations. An even broader perspective calls for studying how the pharmaceutical companies' suppliers themselves obtain their inputs. The supply chain perspective can help pharmaceutical company identify superior suppliers distributors help them improve productivity, which ultimately brings down the company's cost. An efficient supply chain management calls for better materials planning, inventory management, management of transportation and warehouses and also information management.

Market logistics involves planning the infrastructure to meet demand, then implementing and controlling the physical flows of materials and final goods from points of origin to point of use, to meet customer requirement at a profit. Today pharmaceutical companies' worldwide needs logistics management because of competitive pressures, information technology, channel power and profit leverage. Logistics managers are responsible for:

1. Traffic and transportation
2. Materials handling
3. Warehousing and storage
4. Inventory control
5. Order fulfillment
6. Demand forcasting
7. Plant and warehouse site location

Table 3.1 List of price controlled drugs (DPCO 1995)

1. Sulphamethoxazole	22. Salbutamol	43. Pentazocine
2. Penicillins	23. Famotidine	44. Captopril
3. Tetracycline	24. Ibuprofen	45. Naproxen
4. Rifampicin	25. Metamizol (Analgin)	46. Pyrental
5. Streptomycin	26. Doxycycline	47. Sulphadoxine
6. Ranitidine	27. Ciprofloxacin	48. Norfloxacin
7. Vitamin C	28. Cefotaxime	49. Cefadroxyl
8. Betamethasone	29. Dexamethasone	50. Panthonates and Panthenols
9. Metronidazole	30. Ephedrine	51. Furazolidone
10. Chloroquine	31. Vitamin B_1 (Thiamine)	52. Pyrithioxine
11. Insulin	32. Carbamazepine	53. Sulphadiazine
12. Erythromycin	33. Vitamin B_2 (Riboflavin)	54. Framycetin
13. Vitamin A	34. Theophylline	55. Verapamil
14. Oxytetracycline	35. Levodopa	56. Amikacin sulphate
15. Prednisolone	36. Tolnaftate	57. Glipizide
16. Cephazolin	37. Vitamin E	58. Spironolactone
17. Methyldopa	38. Nalidixic Acid	59. Pentoxyfylline
18. Aspirin	39. Griseofulvin	60. Amodiaquin
19. Trimethoprim	40. Gentamicin	
20. Cloxacillin	41. Dextropropoxyphene	
21. Sulphadimidine	42. Halogenated Hydroxyquinoline	

8. Production planning
9. Return good handling.

The major objectives of logistics management

1. To reduce inventory at the minimum possible level.
2. To achieve maximum economy in freight cost.
4. To ensure minimum damage of products during transportation and storage.
5. To ensure quick response to customer requirements.

Logistics Management Decision Areas

1. Transportation
2. Warehousing
3. Inventory

Transportation physically moves products from where they are produced to where they are needed. Transportation moves products to markets which are geographically dispersed and provides added value to customers by transporting products on time, undamaged and in the required quantities. Transportation can impact a firm's ability to exploit a market opportunity. Inadequate transport services, uncertain transit time, and inadequate preparation for transportation, like non-availability of transport permits can lead to a mismatch in demand and supply and hence firms to lead firms in stocking large inventories of finished products. Transportation id major component of logistics cost as and may also account for a significant position for the selling price. For strategic decisions to be made by logistics managers with respect to transportation are:

1. What modes of transportation will the firm use? Will it use road transport, rail transport, water transport, air transport or internodal transportation. Mode of transportation is usually selected on the basis of nature of goods, access to carriers, price, transit time, security of goods, government regulations and safety.
2. What carriers in each mode will the firm use? Carrier selection should be done on the basis of price, accessibility, responsiveness, claims record and reliability.
3. Will the firm operate its own fleet or hire outside carriers for transportation service.
4. Will the firm manage transportation operations or hire a third party?

Transportation accounts for a major portion of the distribution expenditure. The total transportation charges on an average amount to anywhere between 3 to 4% of the sales volume in the case of pharmaceutical companies. In case of companies marketing liquid orals and protein food supplements the transportation costs would be higher than those of marketing ingestible and tablets, etc.

Pharmaceutical companies in India uses road transport mode widely. Infrequently air freight is used only in the case of certain light items like injections and certain life saving drugs where temperature control is a must. Water transportation is used only in the case of exports of pharmaceutical products, since it provides the cheapest way of carrying bulk drugs over a long distance. Many of the companies enter into renewable annual contracts with large transport companies to achieve economy and reliability in terms of safe and speedy delivery.

Warehousing

Every company has to store good until they are sold, because production and consumption cycles rarely match. Major warehousing decision areas are:

1. Number of warehouses and their locations.
2. Level of customer service required to be provided to gain a competitive edge.
3. Own warehouses or third party warehouses.
4. Cost of distribution.
5. Technology to be deployed.

Some of the factors to be considered while locating a depot are: Cost of land, availability of transport, quantity and quality of labour are some of the factors that have to be taken by pharmaceutical firms while taking warehouse decisions.

It is imperative that pharmaceutical products should be stored in warehouses according to GMP standards prescribed by WHO for warehousing as pharmaceutical products are concerned with the health and well-being of human beings. It is important that at all the standards related to the cleanliness temperatures at which the various products are required to be stored are strictly adhered to.

Inventory Management

Inventory levels also impacts the competitive advantage of a firm.

The objectives of inventory management are:

1. To increase corporate profitability through improved inventory management.
2. To predict the impact of corporate policies on inventory levels.
3. To minimize the total cost of logistics activities while making customer service requirements.
4. To avoid out of stock position, because in pharmaceutical marketing it is suicidal as persuading a doctor whose prescription is dishonored once is difficult. This will create a good selling opportunity for the competitors.

Inventory is important because:

1. It enables the firm to achieve economics of scale.
2. It balances supply and demand.

3. It provides protection from uncertainties in demand and order cycle.
4. It acts as a buffer between critical interfaces within the channel of distribution.

Inadequate control of inventories can result in both understocking and overstocking of items. Under stoking results in production hold ups, lost sales, dissatisfied customers, delayed delivery of finished goods, etc. Overstocking unnecessarily ties up working capital funds that might be used more productively elsewhere and also causes inventory carrying cost, obsolescence, wastage due to loss of shelf life, damage in storage, pilferage and so on. Two main concerns of inventory management are:

1. Level of customer service.
2. Cost of ordering and carrying inventories and the shortage costs or stock out costs.

Inventory decision making: Involves knowing when to order and how much to order. For meticulous inventory management companies should follow inventory control Popular inventory control methods are ABC ANALYSIS, Economic Order Quantity, JIT, etc. Q system, P system, X-Y-Z analysis, etc.

Pharmaceutical Pricing

- Price is the total amount of money charged for a product or service. It is the total value that customers exchange for the benefits of having or using products or services.

Objectives of Pricing

- Profit maximization
- Profit optimization
- Assured minimum return on investment or sales turnover
- Ensure a specified targeted sales volume or market share
- Make entry into new markets or achieve deeper market penetration in existing market.
- Maintain price leadership or price parity with competitors
- Launch price war to check competitor's activity or keep competitors out of the race

- Improving cash flow through faster sales
- Liquidation of accumulated inventory of products.

Pricing Strategies

1. *Cost-based pricing:*
   - Mark-up pricing/Cost plus pricing.
   - Absorption cost pricing/Full cost pricing.
   - Target rate of return pricing.
   - Marginal cost pricing.
2. *Demand/market-based pricing:*
   - Skimming pricing.
   - Penetration pricing.
3. *Competition oriented pricing/competition-based pricing/Competetive parity pricing:*
   - Premium pricing.
   - Discount pricing.
   - Parity pricing.
4. Value pricing
5. Product line pricing
6. Tender pricing
7. Affordability-based pricing
8. Differentiated pricing
9. *Psychological pricing:* Hardly any of these methods can be used in pricing pharmaceutical products in India as the prices of a number of bulk drugs and formulations are controlled by the government. There is very little for the pharmaceutical marketer can decide as far as pricing is concerned. Through the input cost are increasing government has put a ceiling on the profits.

NATIONAL PHARMACEUTICAL PRICING AUTHORITY

1. NPPA (National Pharmaceutical Pricing Authority) is an organization of the Government of India which was established, inter alia, to fix/revise the prices of controlled bulk drugs and formulations and to enforce prices and availability of the medicines in the country, under the Drugs (Prices Control) Order, 1995.

2. The organization is also entrusted with the task of recovering amounts overcharged by manufacturers for the controlled drugs from the consumers.
3. It also monitors the prices of decontrolled drugs in order to keep them at reasonable levels.

Functions of National Pharmaceutical Pricing Authority

1. To implement and enforce the provisions of the Drugs (Prices Control) Order in accordance with the powers delegated to it.
2. To deal with all legal matters arising out of the decisions of the Authority;
3. To monitor the availability of drugs, identify shortages, if any, and to take remedial steps;
4. To collect/maintain data on production, exports and imports, market share of individual companies, profitability of companies, etc. for bulk drugs and formulations;
5. To undertake and/or sponsor relevant studies in respect of pricing of drugs/pharmaceuticals;
6. To recruit/appoint the officers and other staff members of the Authority, as per rules and procedures laid down by the Government;
7. To render advice to the central government on changes/revisions in the drug policy;
8. To render assistance to the central government in the parliamentary matters relating to the drug pricing.

INTEGRATED MARKETING COMMUNICATION PHARMACEUTICAL PROMOTION

The marketing communication mix/communication mix/promotion mix consists of the "specific blend of advertising, sales promotion, public relations, personal selling, and direct marketing tools that a company uses to pursue its advertising and marketing objectives".

In marketing, promotion means all those tools that a marketer uses to take his product from the factory to the customer and hence involves advertising, sales promotion, personal selling, public relations, publicity and merchandising. In modern times promotion is also known as marketing communication or integrated marketing communication. The scope of marketing communication or integrated marketing communication is perhaps much wider than promotion. Marketing communications are the means by which firms attempts to inform, persuade, and remind consumers—directly or indirectly about the products and brands that they sell. In a sense, marketing communications represents the voice of the brand and are means by which it can establish a dialogue and build relationships with consumers. Marketing communication perform many functions for consumers. Consumers can be told or shown how any why a product is used, by what kind of person, and where and when, customers can learn about who makes the product and what the company and brand stand for, and consumers can be given an incentive or reward for trial or usage. Marketing communications can contribute to brand equity by establishing the brand in memory and crafting a brand image.

Although advertising is often a central element of a marketing communication programme, it is usually not the only one – or even the most important one—in terms of building brand equity. All communications are action oriented. It is important to note that in the communication process there are two individuals – the sender and the receiver. For communication to be effective, both have to actively involve – the sender in sending message and the receiver in receiving them and giving a feed-back to the sender. In marketing feed-back is in the form of attention paid to a message (commercial, print advertising, salesmen or window display) and actual purchase of the brand being communicated. Getting the receiver (customer) to be interested in his or her message is a major challenge to the marketer. In pharmaceutical marketing almost all tools of Integrated Marketing Communication is targeted at physician, general practitioners, specialist doctors, teaching doctors, dentists, etc. who are the decision makers. In pharmaceutical marketing, personal selling which is a part of personal communication is one of the most potent tools in marketing communication mix. Non-personal communication which includes advertising, sales promotion, publicity and public relations are also often used in promoting pharma products.

The marketing communications mix consists of six major modes of communication.

Advertising

Any paid form of non-personal presentation and promotion of ideas, goods, or services by an identified sponsor.

Objectives of Advertising

- Generating awareness (Informing).
- Creating favorable attitude (Persuasion for attitude formation).
- Managing customer Loyalty (Reinforcement of the desired behaviour).

Tools used for Advertisements

- Print and broadcast ads.
- Packaging outer.
- Packaging inserts.
- Motion pictures.
- Brochures and booklets.
- Posters and leaflets.
- Directories.
- Reprints of ads.
- Billboards.
- Display signs.
- Point-of-purchase displays.
- Audiovisual material.
- Symbols and logos.
- Videotapes.

Advertising in pharmaceutical marketing includes preparation of visual aids, literature medical, product monographs, etc. and advertising in medical journals, souvenirs, print media and commercials for radio and television in case of OTC formulation and preparing advertising material for seminars, medical symposia, etc.

Sales Promotion

Sales promotion consists of short-term incentives to encourage purchase or sales of a product or service. Whereas advertising and personal selling offer reasons to buy a product or service, sales promotion offers reasons to buy now.

Sales Promotion Objectives

a. Increase sales volume
b. Speed up sales for slow moving products
c. Check the fluctuations in sales
d. Attract new customers
e. Launch new products and increase trial
f. Encourage repeat sales
g. Clearance of excessive inventories
h. Motivate dealers
i. Encourage dealers to participate in display and sales contests
j. Gain advantageous shelf-space.

Types of Sales Promotions

- Consumer sales promotions
- Trade promotions
- Business and sales force promotion tools.

Popular Consumer Sales Promotion Tools

1. Samples
2. Coupons
3. Cash refund offers (Rebates)
4. Price packs
5. Premiums (Gifts)
6. Frequency programmes
7. Prizes (contests, sweepstakes, games)
8. Patronage awards
9. Free trials
10. Product warranties
11. Tie-in promotions
12. Cross-promotions
13. Point-of-Purchase (POP) displays and demonstrations.

Trade Promotion Tools

1. Price-off
2. Allowances
3. Free goods.

Business and Sales Force Promotion Tools

1. Trade shows and conventions
2. Sales contests
3. Specialty advertisement

Giving physicians samples and gifts, etc. Special bonus offers, quantity discounts or trade offers free goods and gifts to stockiest and retailers (Gifts to retail chemists on the purchase of predetermined quantity of a product or on value of an assortment of products), etc. are popular sales promotional strategies in pharmaceutical marketing.

Events and Experiences

Company sponsored activities and programmes designs to create daily or special brand–related interactions.

- Sports
- Entertainment
- Festivals
- Arts
- Causes
- Factory tours
- Company museums
- Street activities.

Public Relations and Publicity

A variety of programmes designed to promote or protect a company's image or its individual products. Publicity is the non-personal stimulation of demand for a product, service or business unit by planting commercially significant news about it in a published medium or obtaining favorable presentation of it upon radio, television or stage that is not paid by the sponsor.

- Press kits
- Speeches
- Seminars
- Annual reports
- Charitable donations
- Publications
- Community relations
- Lobbying

- Identity media
- Company magazine.

Organizing medical symposia and seminars, conducting clinical trails, conducting exhibitions, publicity campaigns for innovative products are popular publicity methods in pharmaceutical marketing.

Types of Public Relations

- Media relations
- Employee relations
- Financial relations
- Corporate relations.

Functions of Public Relations

- Helping create a market
- Influencing non consumer groups
- Influencing the influential in crisis
- Influencing the dealers and sales people
- Influencing direct consumers through means other than advertising
- Influencing employees to serve the customers better.

Direct Marketing

Direct Marketing is the use of consumer-direct channels to reach and deliver goods and services to customers without using marketing middlemen. Use of mail, telephone, fax, e-mail, or internet to communicated directly with or solicit response or dialogue from specific customers and prospects. Preparing mailers for doctors and dealers.

Types of Direct Marketing Programmes

1. Direct mail
2. Telemarketing
3. Personal selling
5. Direct response television
6. Direct response print media
7. Direct response radio
8. Database marketing

9. Online marketing
10. Mobile marketing
11. Home shopping shows
12. Personal selling: Personal selling is the direct personal presentation by company sales force for sales and building customer relationship. Face-to-face interaction with one or more prospective purchasers for the purpose of making presentations, answering questions, and procuring orders. In case of pharmaceutical marketing medical representatives details the company's products to doctors with the help of visual aids, literatures, product monographs, etc.

The product's styling and price, the shape and colour of the package, the salesperson's manners and dress, the store decor, the company's stationary all communicate something to buyers. Every brand contact delivers an impression that can strengthen or weaken a customer's view of the company. Marketing communication activities contribute to brand equity in many ways: by creating awareness of the brand, linking the right associations to the brand image in consumer's memory, eliciting positive brand judgements or feelings and/or facilitating a stronger consumer–brand connection. In short it leads to brand awareness, brand image, brand response and brand relationships thus augmenting brand equity.

The Communication Process Model

Communication process models have 9 elements.

- *Sender and • receiver:* Represents the major parties in a communication.
- *Message and • media:* Represents the major communication tools.

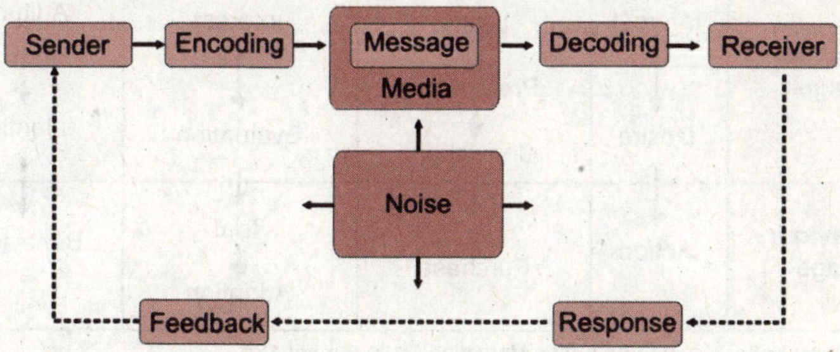

Fig. 3.1: The communication process model

- *Encoding,* • *decoding,* • *response and* • *feedback:* Represents major communication functions.
- *Notice:* Represents random and competing messages that may interfere with the intended communication.

The model emphasizes the key factors in effective communication. Senders must know what audiences they want to reach and what responses they want to get. They must encode there messages so that the target audience can decode them. They must transmit the message through media that reach the target audience and develop feedback channels to monitor the responses. The more the sender's field of experience overlaps with that of the receiver, the more effective the message is likely to be.

Micro model of consumer responses or response hierarchy models:

1. AIDA (Attention-Interest-Desire-Action) model
2. Hierarchy of effects model
3. Innovation-adoption model
4. Communication model.

Micromodel of marketing communications concentrates on consumer's specific responses to communications. All these models

	AIDA Model [a]	Hierarchy of effects Model [b]	Innovation-adoption Model [c]	Communications Model [d]
Cognitive Stage	Attention	Awareness ↓ Knowledge	Awareness	Exposure ↓ Reception ↓ Cognitive Response
Affective Stage	Interest ↓ Desire	Liking ↓ Preference ↓ Conviction	Interest ↓ Evaluation	Attitude ↓ Intention
Behaviour Stage	Action	Purchase	Trial ↓ Adoption	Behaviour

Source: Philip Kotler Kevin Lane Keller *Marketing Management 12e*

Fig. 3.2

assume that the buyer passes through a cognitive, affective and behavioural stage in that order. The "learn-feel –do" sequence is appropriate in pharmaceutical marketing. In short the physician may go through the following stages:

1. *Awareness:* During this stage the physician may be unaware about the product or his attitude may be passive towards the product. If the physician is unaware of the drug, the communicator's task is to build awareness by telling him about the relevant therapeutic category and the particular indication which it is useful for.
2. *Knowledge:* The physician might have brand awareness but not know much more. If knowledge is weak the communicator may decide to select brand knowledge as its communication objective. At this stage the physician is neither passive nor active about the product. By imparting relevant information and key attributes of the product the communicator has to create interest in the doctor's mind.
3. *Liking:* If the physician knows the brand, how does he feel about it? If he looks unfavorably on the brand the communicator must find out why. If the unfavorable view is based on real problems the communicator must fix its problems. Once his doubts are cleared he may include the product in his preference list.
4. *Preference:* The physician might like the product but do not prefer it to others. In this case the communicator must try to build consumer preference by comparing quality, value, preference and other features to likely competitors.
5. *Conviction:* The physician might prefer the product but not have developed a conviction about prescribing it. The communicator's job is to build conviction and prescribing intent.
6. *Evaluation:* The physician may actively consider the product and he will start evaluating the product based on the available information. He will also compare the product with the competitors' products. He will look for the distinct advantages and unique attributes of your product at this stage. Depending upon his needs he will look for safety, enhanced efficacy, economy, reliability, and convenience. At this stage, you have to identify his needs and requirements, increase his confidence by substantiating your product's uniqueness and the ways in which

it would fulfill his needs. You have to make an irresistible presentation of your product benefits and reassure him.

7. *Trial:* After evaluation and convinced about results the physician will move to trial. The communicator at this stage will have to positively reinforce the association between the products unique attributes, the doctor's specific needs and usage opportunities like the indications in which product is most effective.
8. *Prescription:* If the trial is successful the physician will start prescribing the product.
9. *Repeat prescription:* To ensure his continuous prescription support the communicator will have to provide frequent reminders about the product's attributes. Gifts and samples may have to be given at this stage. Usually pharmaceutical companies give gifts where the product name is written and keep it on the table of the doctor for constant reminder. The medical representative has to build up a rapport with the doctor so that he continuously supports the product.

At any given point of time the physician is likely to be at different stages of the buying process. Some may be in the prescribing stage while some others are evaluating the product. Some of them are yet you evince interest in the product. The medical representatives should be capable and alert to understand at which stage the doctor is and take off from that stage.

Developing Effective Marketing Communication

Step 1: Identify the target audience
Step 2: Determine communication objectives
Step 3: Design communication
Step 4: Select channels
Step 5: Establish budget
Step 6: Decide on media mix
Step 7: Measure results
Step 8: Manage intergrated marketing communication.

Effective marketing communication is possible only when the four vital elements are:

1. Source of communication
2. The message

3. The receiver and
4. Feedback are appropriately used. Source credibility, source expertise and source likeability are few factors that are important. The source mix for pharmaceutical companies includes: The company, medical representative, media and trade channels.

Role of advertising in pharmaceutical marketing communication mix: Unlike other product sales, the sales of prescription drug is not based on any choice of the consumer but rather on that of the physician. So prescription medication sales result from derived demand. Prescription drugs are also known as "directed consumer goods". Actually the physicians/doctors constitutes the major "market" for prescription drugs.

Identification of physicians by specialty can be helpful to advertisers in determining the size of the physician audience and in finding the relative use of a product by specialists as opposed to general practitioners, though advertisement is not a powerful promotional tool in pharmaceutical marketing.

So unlike other product advertising which is targeted at the ultimate customer or the user, advertising by pharmaceutical companies are targeted at physicians, general practitioners, specialists, teaching doctors, dentists, etc. The target audience of pharmaceutical advertising is not the ultimate customers or users or beneficiaries of the products. As there are many products in the market place creating top of the mid recall is very important in pharmaceutical advertising. Pharmaceutical advertising includes visual aids for detailing on products by medical representatives, advertising in medical journals, product literatures, monographs and direct mailers. India. Journal advertising and direct mailers are less important as compared to detailing by medicinal representative in pharmaceutical advertising. Preparing a good detailing story is very important in pharmaceutical marketing because it is this story that takes the doctor through different stages of prescription behaviour. An effective detailing story should contain.

1. Detailing story should be built around the single most powerful concept that covers all attribute of the product and benefits that the product can provide to the doctor and his patients.
2. The story should be able to communicate the product benefits creatively, interestingly and differently.

3. The detailing story should be memorable so that your product receives top of the mind recall in an overcrowded market place. The colours and pictures used should be appealing and eye-catching.
4. The main concept and the brand name should be repeated often.
5. The medical representative can use AIDA formula to be one effective in communication the idea.

Examples of some good visual aids to be included

Role of personal selling in pharmaceutical marketing communicating mix: Pharmaceutical industry in India is characterized by intense competition as there are more than 23,000 pharmaceutical companies. So personal selling is one of the most vital tools used by pharmaceutical companies to promote their products. Thus personal selling and quality of sales force emerges as crucial determinants of success in the pharmaceutical marketing. Though personal selling is an important element for selling mutual funds, insurance, industrial goods and FMCG, their personal selling efforts are supported by mass media advertising and other equally potent promotional tools. Role of intermediaries are limited in selling of these products. There marketing strategies targets the ultimate user or the end customer. Whereas, in pharmaceutical marketing mass media advertising plays a very minor role or even no role is played by it. Pharmaceutical marketer's target is not the patients or the ultimate customers or end users, but the physicians or the intermediary who prescribes, recommends and advises the product to the end users. The law of the land which does not permit the patients to purchase medicines without the prescription of physicians coupled with the technical nature of the product forces the patient to take the help of a physician. On the other hand the most major source of information for the doctor is interaction with the medical representative, who details the company's products to doctors, with the help of visual aids, leave behind literature, product monographs, samples, gifts, etc. The medical representative through his selling skills and product knowledge will have to convince the doctor to prescribe his product.

Personal selling is an ancient art and a powerful tool of marketing communication. Today in a world marked by standardization of technology leading to undifferentiated products it is a sales person through personal selling who provide competitive advantage to an enterprise as it is he or she who services the customer. The customer knows the firm through the salesperson. Hence it is the quality of selling and the relationship that a salesperson builds with he customer that gives the enterprise competitive edge. It may be noted that personal selling is the most important determinant factor of success of pharmaceutical marketing as pharmaceutical marketing is highly specialized. As well as the role of mass advertising in pharmaceutical marketing is limited, prescription of a registered doctor.

The sales persons in pharmaceutical marketing are usually known as medical representatives. Medical representatives are responsible for meeting doctors and persuading or convincing them to write his company product. Successful Medical representatives should have some qualities like,

1. Product knowledge
2. Good communication skills
3. Pleasant manners and appearance
4. Confidence.

Sales person and five types of knowledge:

1. Know the company
2. Know the competition
3. Know the customer
4. Know the selling process
5. Know own self.

Personality traits required by a good medical representative:

1. Dominance
2. Achiever
3. Affiliation
4. Creativity
5. Flamboyant
6. Problem solving.

Role of a medical representative:

1. Diagnostic
2. Analyst
3. Information provider

4. Strategist
5. Tactician
6. Change agent.

Major steps involved in sales process:

1. Prospecting and qualifying
2. Pre-approach
3. Presentation and demonstration
4. Overcoming objections
5. Closing
6. Follow-up and maintenance.

Tasks performed by medical representatives: A medical representative has to perform the following tasks. His success in his career also depends on how well he is able to perform these tasks.

1. ***Detailing to doctors:*** The products have to be explained to the doctor. For this salesman should carry a detailing book which covers the salient features of all the company products. The medical representative should be well equipped with minute details of the product and even competitor's products while detailing. The MR can also use product brochures for this purpose.
2. ***Sampling to doctors:*** After detailing samples have to be provided to the doctor. The doctor may use the samples for trials, or give it to poor patients or simply keep in his table as reminder.
3. ***Monitoring sales:*** Sales of his territory has to be monitored on a day to day basis. This can be done with the help of stockiest, distributors and retailers. If he finds that the sales is down immediately the MR can start aggressive selling or meeting doctors and reminding about products.
4. ***Retailing:*** Stockiest and chemists have to be visited regularly. It gives vital feedback on what is happening to your products and how they are moving. Competitors activities their products movements, their future plans, identification of major prescribers of your products as well as your competitor's basic information leading to effective prospecting.

Role of sales promotion in integrated pharmaceutical marketing communication: The sales promotion methods used in pharmaceutical marketing are:

a. Discounts on quantity purchased

b. Trade offers
c. Gifts to retail chemists on the basis of quantity purchased or on value of purchase as fixed by pharmaceutical companies periodically.

PROMOTIONAL TOOLS AND PHYSICIANS

Physicians are the most important factor in pharmaceutical marketing. The pharmaceutical product—The drugs can be sold to the ultimate customer, only if the physician prescribes. Physicians are keen to know about drugs, old or new. There are hundreds and thousands of medicines in the market and many are launched daily. The information about a drug is provided by a pharma company, through its medical representatives. Physicians are primarily interested in patient care and information about scientific advances. So they should be provided with information about the particular product, its competitive advantage with respect to the competing product, and also with scientific advances in the particular field. Just passing on this information does not work for the favour of the particular company in pharmaceutical marketing. The success depends on whether the physician prescribes the product or not. So influencing the physician is key to pharmaceutical sales. Pharmaceutical companies try to influence prescription pattern of doctors in favour of their brands by offering various kinds of promotional inputs like samples, gifts and sponsorships, etc. Pharmaceutical companies interact with the doctors through their team of medical representatives, area managers and regional managers. The frequency of a medical representative's meeting a doctor depends on the quantum of his contribution in terms of prescription volume. Medical representatives meet busy practitioners at least 4 times a month. In advanced countries a doctor receives on an average 6 gifts with an average value of $60 per year. Expensive gifts are also given to doctors. Physicians travel expenses, sometimes families, stay and local sight seeing are paid directly to the tour operator by the pharmaceutical company or travel ticket and hotel accommodation are booked by the company in the name of the physician. The most common promotional inputs pharmaceutical companies include are: (a) Offering vacation/travel expenses; (b) Gifts of substantial value; (c) Lavish meals and entertainment; (d) Offering cash/commission for prescribing a particular brand/drug; (e)

Offering money for drug trial; (f) Samples and promotional material; and (g) CME funding and honoraria. Pharmaceutical companies spend huge amount of money in interacting and influencing the physicians. This sales strategy employed by the pharmaceutical industry bolsters their bottom lines, and is done in a planned process. Studies reveal that sponsorships, either for personal or professional purpose, have been one of the most influencing factors to increase prescription rates of the sponsor's products. Some physicians give more importance to product literature/updates; textbooks, etc. whereas a third category of doctors perceived that visits by medical representative with pleasing personality and good product knowledge are best tools of promotion.

As the objective of modern marketing is to make profits through satisfying customer needs and wants, the marketers have to understand the real needs, wants, beliefs and attitudes of customers towards products and services. Physicians being the most important players in pharmaceutical sales, write the prescriptions that determine which drugs will be used by the patient. Influencing the physician is key to pharmaceutical sales and using appropriate promotional tools company can perform better than the competitors.

ADVERTISING BUDGET

1. Percentage of sales volume
2. Unit of sales method
3. Competitive parity method
4. Historical method
5. Affordability method
6. Total group budget
7. Percentage of anticipated turnover
8. Elasticity method
9. Operational modelling
10. Composite method
11. Objective and task method.

4 Conclusion

FUTURE PROSPECTS

As per WTO, from the year 2005, India will grant product patent recognition to all new chemical entities (NCEs), i.e. bulk drugs developed then onwards. The Indian Government's decision to allow 100% foreign direct investment into the drugs and pharmaceutical industry is expected to aid the growth of contract research in the country. Technology transfer to 100% Indian subsidiaries of MNCs is expected only in 2005.

ADVANTAGE INDIA

Competent workforce: India has a pool of personnel with high managerial and technical competence as also skilled workforce. It has an educated work force and English is commonly used. Professional services are easily available.

Costeffective chemical synthesis: Its track record of development, particularly in the area of improved cost-beneficial chemical synthesis for various drug molecules is excellent. It provides a wide variety of bulk drugs and exports sophisticated bulk drugs.

Legal and financial framework: India has a 53-year and old democracy and hence has a solid legal framework and strong financial markets. There is already an established international industry and business community.

Information and technology: It has a good network of world-class educational institutions and established strengths in Information Technology.

Globalization: The country is committed to a free market economy and globalization. Above all, it has a 70 million middle class market, which is continuously growing.

Consolidation: For the first time in many years, the international pharmaceutical industry is finding great opportunities in India. The process of consolidation, which has become a generalized phenomenon in the world pharmaceutical industry, has started taking place in India.

Steps to Strengthen the Industry

Indian companies need to attain the right product-mix for sustained future growth. Core competencies will play an important role in determining the future of many Indian pharmaceutical companies in the post product-patent regime after 2005. Indian companies, in an effort to consolidate their position, will have to increasingly look at merger and acquisition options of either companies or products. This would help them to offset loss of new product options, improve their R&D efforts and improve distribution to penetrate markets.

Research and development has always taken the back seat amongst Indian pharmaceutical companies. In order to stay competitive in the future, Indian companies will have to refocus and invest heavily in R&D.

The Indian pharmaceutical industry also needs to take advantage of the recent advances in biotechnology and information technology. The future of the industry will be determined by how well it markets its products to several regions and distributes risks, its forward and backward integration capabilities, its R&D, its consolidation through mergers and acquisitions, co-marketing and licensing agreements.

Indian pharmaceutical interests in making a mark on the global scene got a boost when Dr Reddy's licensed two of its anti-diabetic molecules to Novo Nordisk and when Ranbaxy licensed its Novel Drug Delivery System (NDDS) of ciprofloxacin to Bayer. MNCs in India faced the problem of having a very high Drug Price Control Order (DPCO) coverage, weakening their bottom lines as well as hindering their growth through the launch of new products. DPCO coverage is expected to be diluted further in the near future benefiting the MNCs. New legislation is also expected in the OTC segment increasing the number of brands in the Over the Counter (OTC) segment.

The Indian pharmaceutical industry is also getting increasingly US FDA compliant to harness the growth opportunities in areas of contract manufacturing and research. Indian companies such as Ranbaxy, Sun Pharma, and Dr Reddy's are increasingly focusing on tapping the US generic market, projected to be around $18 billion by 2004.

Research and Development

Research and Development is the key to the future of pharmaceutical industry. The pharmaceutical advances for considerable improvement in life expectancy and health all over the world are the result of a steadily increasing investment in research. There is considerable scope for collaborative R&D in India. India can offer several strengths to the international R&D community. These strengths relate to availability of excellent scientific talents who can develop combinatorial chemistry, new synthetic molecules and plant derived candidate drugs.

R&D in the pharmaceutical industry in India is critical to find answers for some of the diseases peculiar to a tropical country like India and also for finding solutions for unmet medical needs. Industrial R&D groups can carry out limited primary screening to identify lead molecules or even candidate drugs for further *in vivo* screening, pre-clinical pharmacology, toxicology, animal and human pharmacokinetics and metabolic studies before taking them up for human trials. In such collaborations, harmonized standards of screening can be assured following established good laboratory practices.

The R&D expenditure by the Indian pharmaceutical industry is around 1.9% of the industry's turnover. This obviously, is very low when compared to the investment on R&D by foreign research-based pharma companies. They spend 10–16% of the turnover on R&D. However, now that India is entering into the Patent protection area, many companies are spending relatively more on R&D.

When it comes to clinical evaluation at the time of multi-center trials, India would provide a strong base considering the real availability of clinical materials in diverse therapeutic areas. Such active collaboration will be mutually beneficial to both partners. According to a survey by the Pharmaceutical Outsourcing Management Association and Bio/Pharmaceutical Outsourcing Report, pharmaceutical companies are utilizing substantially the services of Contract Research Organizations (CROs).

Indian Pharmaceutical Industry, with its rich scientific talents, provides cost effective clinical trial research. It has an excellent record of development of improved, cost-beneficial chemical syntheses for various drug molecules. Some MNCs are already sourcing these services from their Indian affiliates.

The Pharmaceutical and Biotechnology Industry is eligible for weight deduction for R&D expense up to 150%. These R&D companies will also enjoy tax holiday for 10 years. A promotional research and development fund of Rs 150 crores is set-up by the Government to promote research and development in the pharmaceuticals sector.

Key Findings

- The domestic pharmaceutical market in India has grown at a CAGR of nearly 12% in the last five years.
- At present, drugs for mass therapies dominate, however, driven by an increasing prevalence of lifestyle-associated diseases, drugs for specialty therapies are expected to remain buoyant in future.
- Around 67 million Indians are expected to be above 67 years of age by 2011. This age group spends around 3 to 4 times more on drugs than those in younger age groups, thus fuelling the market growth.
- Patented drugs, which had no share in the pharmaceutical market, are expected to have a 10% market share in 2010.
- Around 64% Indians are not covered under by health insurance and pay expenses for pharmaceuticals out of pocket.

Driven by factors such as rising rural incomes and a strong distribution network, India's rural pharmaceutical market is experiencing a strong growth.

Employment Opportunities in Pharmaceutical Sector

The demand for a skilled workforce to power this sector now presents unprecedented employment opportunities for aspirants.

Research and Development

Research and development has several areas like drug discovery which is discovery of new molecule. R&D can deal with the development of generic products, analytical R&D, API (Active Pharmaceutical Ingredients) or bulk drugs R&D, or development of formulations, etc. R&D also can deal with drug delivery, which can be in the form of a tablet, capsule or injection.

Quality Control

Quality Control is a very critical function of the pharmaceutical industry. Besides researching and developing new drugs, there is also a need to ensure that drugs can be marketed as those that produce results, which are safe, consistent and predictable.

Manufacturing

Manufacturing pertains to actual production of the drug. The aspirant can either be involved in API manufacturing, while someone with a pharmacy background, can also build a career in manufacturing formulations.

Clinical Research

Screening of drugs involves testing new drugs or formulations on animal models or conducting clinical research, which is essentially human testing. Clinical research has recently witnessed international interest with foreign companies coming to India to conduct clinical research.

Regulation

Pharma is a regulated industry the world over, and professionals who can manage regulatory affairs, are in high demand.

Registered Pharmacist

Unlike in India, pharmacists abroad have a very important role. Just like a doctor would require a license to practice pharmacy, they have to require a license to practice pharmacy. They have to pass a test to register themselves. This is a very lucrative job abroad.

The Pharmacy Council of India has started a six-year programme, Pharm D, to provide training in this discipline.

Sales and Marketing

A person with a B Pharm with an MBA degree can peruse a career in sales and marketing as marketing is extremely important in the pharmaceutical sector. A marketing professional deals with selling, competition mapping, and determining which product has more potential and the strategy for the product.

Other Options

Customer Research and Manufacturing (CRAM) is a booming area as many foreign pharma companies outsource their manufacturing to India.

Pharma students can also work with NGOs involved in public health, like the Rural Health Commission.

There are also opportunities in finance, supply chain, human resources, IT and legal, for which respective education in the respective domains is required. Most of the good companies have a legal unit with professionals who determine whether a drug the company is planning to develop is patentable.

Remuneration: Depending on one's qualification, the institute, and the company that is hiring a postgraduate can expect a minimum of 2–3 lakhs/annum and a maximum of 9 lakhs per annum.

Government Policies

1. Pharmaceutical Policy 2002
2. Drugs Price Control Order (DPCO)

PHARMACEUTICAL POLICY 2002

Intoduction

The basic objectives of Government's Policy relating to the drugs and pharmaceutical sector were enumerated in the Drug Policy of 1986. These basic objectives still remain largely valid. However, the drug and pharmaceutical industry in the country today faces new challenges on account of liberalization of the Indian economy, the globalization of the world economy and on account of new obligations undertaken by India under the WTO Agreements. These challenges require a change in emphasis in the current pharmaceutical policy and the need for new initiatives beyond those enumerated in the Drug Policy 1986, as modified in 1994, so that policy inputs are directed more towards promoting accelerated growth of the pharmaceutical industry and towards making it more internationally competitive. The need for radically improving the policy framework for knowledge-based industry has also been acknowledged by the Government. The Prime Minister's Advisory Council on Trade and Industry has made important recommendations regarding knowledge-based industry. The pharmaceutical industry has been identified as one of the most important knowledge based industries in which India has a comparative advantage.

The process of liberalization set in motion in 1991, has considerably reduced the scope of industrial licensing and demolished many non-tariff barriers to imports. Important steps already taken in this regard are:

- Industrial licensing for the manufacture of all drugs and pharmaceuticals has been abolished except for bulk drugs produced by the use of recombinant DNA technology, bulk drugs requiring *in vivo* use of nucleic acids, and specific cell/tissue targeted formulations.
- Reservation of 5 drugs for manufacture by the public sector only was abolished in Feb.1999, thus opening them up for manufacture by the private sector also.
- Foreign investment through automatic route was raised from 51 to 74% in March, 2000 and the same has been raised to 100%.
- Automatic approval for Foreign Technology Agreements is being given in the case of all bulk drugs, their intermediates and formulations except those produced by the use of recombinant DNA technology, for which the procedure prescribed by the Government would be followed.
- Drugs and pharmaceuticals manufacturing units in the public sector are being allowed to face competition including competition from imports. Wherever possible, these units are being privatized.

- Extending the facility of weighted deductions of 150% of the expenditure on in-house research and development to cover as eligible expenditure, the expenditure on filing patents, obtaining regulatory approvals and clinical trials besides R&D in biotechnology.
- Introduction of the Patents (Second Amendment) bill in the Parliament. It, inter-alia, provides for the extension in the life of a patent to 20 years.

The impact of the policies enunciated, from time to time, by the Government has been salutary. It has enabled the pharmaceutical industry to meet almost entirely the country's demand for formulations and substantially for bulk drugs. In the process the pharmaceutical industry in India has achieved global recognition as a low cost producer and supplier of quality bulk drugs and formulations to the world. In 1999-2000, drugs and pharmaceutical exports were Rs. 6631 crores out of a total production of Rs. 19,737 crores. However, two major issues have surfaced on account of globalization and implementation of our obligations under Trips which impact on long-term competitiveness of Indian industry. These have been addressed in the Pharmaceutical Policy 2002. A reorientation of the objectives of the current policy has also become necessary on account of these issues:

a. The essentiality of improving incentives for research and development in the Indian pharmaceutical industry, to enable the industry to achieve sustainable growth particularly in view of anticipated changes in the Patent Law; and
b. The need for reducing further the rigour of price control particularly in view of the ongoing process of liberalization.

It is against this backdrop, that Pharmaceutical Policy 2002 is being enunciated.

Objectives

The main objectives of this policy are:

a. Ensuring abundant availability at reasonable prices within the country of good quality essential pharmaceuticals of mass consumption.

b. Strengthening the indigenous capability for cost effective quality production and exports of pharmaceuticals by reducing barriers to trade in the pharmaceutical sector.
c. Strengthening the system of quality control over drug and pharmaceutical production and distribution to make quality an essential attribute of the Indian pharmaceutical industry and promoting rational use of pharmaceuticals.
d. Encouraging R&D in the pharmaceutical sector in a manner compatible with the country's needs and with particular focus on diseases endemic or relevant to India by creating an environment conducive to channelising a higher level of investment into R&D in pharmaceuticals in India.
e. Creating an incentive framework for the pharmaceutical industry which promotes new investment into pharmaceutical industry and encourages the introduction of new technologies and new drugs.

Approach adopted in the review:

1. In order to strengthen the pharmaceutical industry's research and development capabilities and to identify the support required by Indian pharmaceutical companies to undertake domestic R&D, a Committee was set up in 1999 by this Department by the name of Pharmaceutical Research and Development Committee (PRDC) under the Chairmanship of Director General of CSIR.
2. To qualify as R&D intensive company in India, the PRDC has suggested following conditions (gold standards):
   - Invest at least 5% of its turnover per annum in R&D,
   - Invest at least Rs.10 crore per annum in innovative research including new drug development, new delivery systems, etc. in India,
   - Employ at least 100 research scientists in R&D in India,
   - Has been granted at least 10 patents for research done in India,
   - Own and operate manufacturing facilities in India.
3. The recommendations of the PRDC in so far as they relate to the Pharmaceutical Policy have been taken into account while formulating the proposals on pricing aspects.
4. The Pharmaceutical Research and Development Committee has recommended in its report, submitted inter-alia, the setting up

of a Drug Development Promotion Foundation (DDPF) and a Pharmaceutical Research and Development Support Fund (PRDSF). Necessary action in this regard has been initiated.

5. As far as the question of price control is concerned, the span of control has been gradually reduced since 1979. Presently, under DPCO, 1995 there are 74 bulk drugs and their formulations under price control covering approximately 40% of the total market. The functioning of the Drugs (Price Control) Order, 1995, has brought to light some problems in the administration of the price control mechanism for drugs and pharmaceuticals. In order to review the current drug price control mechanism, with the objective, inter-alia, of reducing the rigour of price control, where they have become counter-productive, a committee, called the Drugs Price Control Review Committee (DPCRC), under the Chairmanship of Secretary, Department of Chemicals and Petrochemicals was set up in 1999, which has given its report. The recommendations of DPCRC have been examined and taken into account while formulating the "Pharmaceutical Policy 2002".
6. It has emerged that the domestic drugs and pharmaceuticals industry needs reorientation in order to meet the challenges and harness opportunities arising out of the liberalization of the economy and the impending advent of the product patent regime. It has been decided that the span of price control over drugs and pharmaceuticals would be reduced substantially. However, keeping in view the interest of the weaker sections of the society, it is proposed that the Government will retain the power to intervene comprehensively in cases where prices behave abnormally.
7. In view of the steps already taken and in the light of the approach indicated in the foregoing paragraphs, the decisions of the Government are detailed below:

Industrial Licensing

Industrial licensing for all bulk drugs cleared by Drug Controller General (India), all their intermediates and formulations will be abolished, subject to stipulations laid down from time to time in the Industrial Policy, except in the cases of:

i. Bulk drugs produced by the use of recombinant DNA technology,
ii. Bulk drugs requiring *in vivo* use of nucleic acids as the active principles, and
iii. Specific cell/tissue targeted formulations.

Foreign Investment

Foreign investment up to 100% will be permitted, subject to stipulations laid down from time to time in the Industrial Policy, through the automatic route in the case of all bulk drugs cleared by Drug Controller General (India), all their intermediates and formulations, except those, referred to in para 12. I above, kept under industrial licensing.

Foreign Technology Agreements

Automatic approval for Foreign Technology Agreements will be available in the case of all bulk drugs cleared by Drug Controller General (India), all their intermediates and formulations, except those, referred to in para 12. I above, kept under industrial licensing for which a special procedure prescribed by the Government would be followed.

Imports

Imports of drugs and pharmaceuticals will be as per EXIM policy in force. A centralized system of registration will be introduced under the Drugs and Cosmetics Act and Rules made there under. Ministry of Health and Family Welfare will enforce strict regulatory processes for import of bulk drugs and formulations.

Encouragement to Research and Development (R&D)

a. In principle approval to the establishment of the Pharmaceutical Research and Development Support Fund (PRDSF) under the administrative control of the Department of Science and Technology, which will also constitute a Drug Development Promotion Board (DDPB) on the lines of the Technology Development Board to administer the utilization of the PRDSF.

b. With a view to encouraging generation of intellectual property and facilitating indigenous endeavors in Pharma R&D, appropriate fiscal incentives would be provided.

Pricing

Span of Price Control: The guiding principle for identification of specific bulk drugs for price regulation should continue, as per DPCRC's recommendation, to be: (a) Mass consumption nature of the drug and (b) absence of sufficient competition in such drugs. However, the DPCRC's recommendation regarding the new criteria for ascertaining the mass consumption nature of a bulk drug on the basis of the top selling brand is not acceptable as it gives rise to anomalies.

In this context, it may be noted that there is no tailor made data available for the purpose of ascertaining the mass consumption nature and absence of sufficient competition with reference to a particular bulk drug. There is only one source namely, "Retail Store Audit for Pharmaceutical Market in India" published by ORG-MARG, which lists out all major brands and their sale estimates on All India basis. This publication contains data for single ingredient as well as multi-ingredient formulations. However, it does not give complete description of all the ingredients of the pharmaceutical product listed therein.

Hence, there is need to obtain information in regard to composition of each brand, dosage formwise and packwise, from various other publications/sources, viz.

a. Indian Pharmaceutical Guide (IPG)

- Current Index of Medical Specialities (CIMS)
- Monthly Index of Medical Specialities (MIMS)
- Drug today
- Information provided by some manufacturers
- Label composition as indicated on market samples.

Though none of these sources can be said to be exhaustive and comprehensive in regard to market information, yet under the given circumstances, these are the best available. It has also been noted that the sale value of any combination formulation is not directly relatable to a single particular bulk drug forming part of the combination formulation. Combination formulations involve too many variables, viz., strength of a particular bulk drug and its proportion with respect to other bulk drugs used in the combination formulation, price difference between bulk drugs used in combination formulation, pack sizes, dosage forms, etc. In view of these facts, ORG-MARG sales data for combination formulations does not yield information in regard to mass consumption nature and absence of sufficient competition with reference to a particular bulk drug. Also, it is to be borne in mind that processing of such data, which requires cross-checking with other publications and sources of information in regard to composition of each brand, dosage form-wise and pack-wise may involve instances of omission/commission.

In view of above, it would be logical to conclude that although ORG-MARG sale estimates available in regard to all single-ingredient formulations of a particular bulk drug would not yield the sale value of that bulk drug in the form of all its formulations, yet it would adequately reflect the mass consumption nature of that bulk drug in the form of single ingredient formulations, which may be used as a practical indicator for formulating the policy.

The department through NPPA, with the help of NIPER has developed the desired database for single ingredient formulations from the retail store audit data as published by ORG-MARG. On this basis, the Department proposes to undertake the exercise of identifying the bulk drugs of mass consumption nature and having absence of sufficient competition according to the following methodology:

i. The 279 items appearing in the alphabetical list of Essential Drugs in the National Essential Drug List (1996) of the Ministry of Health and Family Welfare and the 173 items, which are considered important by that Ministry from the point of view of their use in various Health Programmes, in emergency care, etc. with the exclusion. as in the past, there from of sera and vaccines, blood products, combinations, etc. should form the total basket out of which selection of bulk drugs be made for price regulation.

ii. The ORG-MARG data of March 2001 would form the basis for determining the span of price control as suggested by DPCRC.

iii. The Moving Annual Total (MAT) value for any formulator in respect of any bulk drug will be arrived at by adding the MAT values of all his single-ingredient formulations of that bulk drug, its salts, esters, stereo-isomers and derivatives, covering all the strengths, dosage forms and pack sizes listed against that formulator in all groups/categories of the ORG-MARG (March 2001).

iv. The MAT value for all the formulators, as defined in sub-para (iii) above, in respect of a particular bulk drug will be added to arrive at the total MAT value in the retail trade.

v. The MAT value for an individual formulator, in respect of any bulk drug, as arrived at in sub-para (iii) above, will be the basis for calculating the percentage share of that formulator in the total MAT value arrived at as in sub-para (iv) above, in respect of that bulk drug.

vi. Bulk drugs will be kept under price regulation if:

- The total MAT value, arrived at as in sub-para (iv) above, in respect of any particular bulk drug is more than Rs. 2500 lakes (Rs. 25 crores) and the percentage share, as defined in sub-para (v) above, of any of the formulators is 50% or more.
- The total MAT value, arrived at as in sub-para (iv) above, in respect of any particular bulk drug is less than Rs. 2500 lakes (Rs. 25 cores) but more than Rs. 1000 lakes (Rs. 10 crores) and the percentage share, as defined in sub-para (v) above, of any of the formulators is 90% or more.

vii. All formulations containing a bulk drug as identified above, either individually or in combination with other bulk drugs, including those not identified for price control as bulk drug, will be under price control. The Government shall, however, retain the following over-riding power:

In cases of drugs/formulations listed by the Ministry of Health and Family Welfare, mentioned in sub-para (i) above, and those presently under price control, having significant MAT value as per ORG-MARG but not covered under the criteria in sub-para (vi) above, as a result of this proposal, the NPPA would specially monitor intensively their price movement and consumption pattern. If any unusual movement of prices is observed or brought to the notice of the NPPA, the Authority would work out the price in accordance with the relevant provisions of the price control order.

b. Maximum Allowable Post-manufacturing Expenses (MAPE):

Maximum Allowable Post-manufacturing Expenses (MAPE) will be 100% for indigenously manufactured formulations.

c. Margin for Imported Formulations

For imported formulations, the margin to cover selling and distribution expenses including interest and importer's profit shall not exceed fifty percent of the landed cost.

d. Pricing of Formulations

- For Scheduled formulations, prices shall be determined as per the present practice. The time frame for granting price approvals will be two months from the date of the receipt of the complete prescribed information.
- The present stipulation that a manufacturer, distributor or wholesaler shall sell a formulation to a retailer, unless otherwise permitted under the provisions of Drugs (Prices Control) Order or any other order made there under, at a price equal to the retail price, as specified by an order or notified by the Government, (excluding excise duty, if any) minus sixteen percent thereof in case of Scheduled drugs, will continue.
- The present provision of limiting profitability of pharmaceutical companies, as per the Third Schedule of the present Drugs (Prices Control) Order, 1995, would be done away with. However, if necessary so to do in public interest, price of any formulation including a non-scheduled formulation would be fixed or revised by the Government.

e. Ceiling Prices

Ceiling prices may be fixed for any formulation, from time to time and it would be obligatory for all, including small scale units or those marketing under generic name, to follow the price so fixed.

f. Exemptions

- A manufacturer producing a new drug patented under the Indian Patent Act, 1970, and not produced elsewhere, if developed through indigenous R&D, would be eligible for exemption from price control in respect of that drug for a period of 15 years from the date of the commencement of its commercial production in the country.

- A manufacturer producing a drug in the country by a process developed through indigenous R&D and patented under the Indian Patent Act, 1970, would be eligible for exemption from price control in respect of that drug till the expiry of the patent from the date of the commencement of its commercial production in the country by the new patented process.
- A formulation involving a new delivery system developed through indigenous R&D and patented under the Indian Patent Act, 1970, for process patent for formulation involving new delivery system would be eligible for exemption from price control in favour of the patent holder formulator from the date of the commencement of its commercial production in the country till the expiry of the patent.
- The DPCRC has suggested that the low cost drugs measured in terms of "cost per day per medicine" may be taken out of price control. Any formulator can represent to NPPA with proof of per day cost to consumer-patient. NPPA will be authorized to exempt such formulation from price control if its cost to consumer-patient does not exceed Rs. 2 per day, under intimation to the Government. All orders passed by the NPPA will be prospective in operation. Whenever the concerned formulator wishes to revise the price, he, before effecting any change in price, would be bound to inform NPPA and seek fresh exemption and in case the cost to consumer-patient, on the basis of the proposed revised price, exceeds beyond the limit of Rs. 2 per day, obtain the necessary price approval.

g. Pricing of Scheduled Bulk Drugs

- For a Scheduled bulk drug, the rate of return in case of basic manufacture would be higher by 4% over the existing 14% on net worth or 22% on capital employed. The time frame for granting price approvals will be 4 months from the date of the receipt of the complete prescribed information.
- The Government shall, however, retain the overriding power of fixing the maximum sale price of any bulk drug, in public interest.

h. Monitoring

- The DPCRC's recommendations to have effective monitoring and enforcement system and to move away from the "controlled regime" to a "monitoring regime" is in the present context an extremely important recommendation as imports will increasingly compete with local drugs and pharmaceuticals in the domestic market. A new system based on solely market prices data is required to be evolved and controls applied selectively only to cases where, either profiteering or monopoly profit seeking is noticed. The National Pharmaceutical Pricing Authority, set up in August, 1997, would need to be revamped and reoriented for this purpose. It will continue to be entrusted with the task of price fixation/price revision and other related matters, and would be empowered to take final decisions. It would also monitor the prices of decontrolled drugs and formulations and over-see the implementation of the drug prices control orders. The Government would have the power of review of the price fixation/and price revision orders/notifications of NPPA.

- Although the prices of some bulk drugs have been steadily decreasing, yet the same do not get reflected in the retail price of non-Scheduled formulations. Also, there is need to check high margin/commission offered to the trade by printing high prices on the labels of medicines to the detriment of the consumers. It is, therefore, proposed to strengthen the National Pharmaceutical Pricing Authority (NPPA) by providing appropriate powers under the DPCO which would make it mandatory for the manufacturer to furnish all information as called for by NPPA and also to regulate such prices, wherever, required.
- The other recommendations of DPCRC like giving powers to drug control authorities to dispose of small and petty offences, etc. will require an amendment to the Essential Commodities Act. This suggestion is considered not practicable. Monitoring price movement of drugs sold in the country as well as that of imported formulations will require developing appropriate mechanism in the NPPA.

i. Drug Price Equalization Account (DPEA)

Provision would be made in the new Drugs Prices Control Order (DPCO) to ensure that amounts which have already accrued to the DPEA and those which are likely to accrue as a result of action in the past, are protected and used for the purpose stipulated in the existing DPCO.

Quality Aspects

The Ministry of Health and Family Welfare would

i. Progressively benchmark the regulatory standards against the international standards for manufacturing,
ii. Progressively harmonize standards for clinical testing with international practices,
iii. Streamline the procedures and steps for quick evaluation and clearance of new drug applications, developed in India through indigenous R&D, and
iv. Set up a world class Central Drug Standard Control Organisation (CDSCO) by modernizing, restructuring and reforming the existing system and establish an effective net work of drugs standards enforcement administrations in the States with the CDSCO as a nodal center, to ensure high standards of quality, safety and efficacy of drugs and pharmaceuticals.

Pharma Education and Training

The National Institute of Pharmaceutical Education and Research (NIPER) have been set up by the Government of India as an institute of "national importance" to achieve excellence in pharmaceutical sciences and technologies, education and training. Through this institute, Government's endeavor will be to upgrade the standards of pharmacy education and R&D. Besides tackling problems of human resources development for academic and the indigenous pharmaceutical industry, the institute will make efforts to maximize collaborative research with the industry and other technical institutes in the area of drug discovery and pharma technology development.

DRUGS PRICE CONTROL ORDER (DPCO)

Drugs and formulations have been subjected to price control for more than three decades now. The economic reforms initiated by the Government of India in July 1991, trickled down to the Pharmaceutical Industry only in 1994 and that too partially. Price control in a large number of industries has already been abolished.

The main objectives of the Drug Policy after the modifications in the Policy of 1986 announced in September 1994 are to ensure availability, at reasonable prices of essential and life saving and prophylactic medicines of good quality; strengthening the system of quality control over drug production and promoting the rational use of drugs in the country; creating an environment conducive for channelising new investment into the pharmaceutical industry to encourage costeffective production with economic sizes and introducing new technologies and new drugs; and strengthening the indigenous capability for production of drugs.

The Drugs Price Control Order (DPCO), 1995 is an order issued by the Government of India under Section 3 of the Essential Commodities Act, 1955 to regulate the prices of drugs. The Order inter alia provides the list of price controlled drugs, procedures for fixation of prices of drugs, method of implementation of prices fixed by Government and penalties for contravention of provisions among other things. For the purpose of implementing provisions of DPCO, powers of the Government have been vested in the National Pharmaceutical Pricing Authority (NPPA). Drugs are essential for health of the society. Drugs have been declared as essential and accordingly put under the Essential Commodities Act. Only 74 out of 500 commonly used bulk drugs are kept under statutory price control. All formulations containing these bulk drugs either in a single or combination form fall under the price control category. However, the prices of other drugs can be regulated, if warranted in public interest.

The NPPA was established on 29th August 1997 as an independent body of experts following the Cabinet Committee's decision in September 1994 while reviewing the Drug Policy. The Authority, inter alia, has been entrusted with the task of fixation/ revision of prices of pharmaceutical products (bulk drugs and formulations), enforcement of provisions of the Drugs (Prices Control) Order and monitoring the prices of controlled and decontrolled drugs in the country.

Various Pharmaceutical Associations

1. **Indian Drug Manufacturers Association**
   102-B, Poonam Chambers, A-Wing,
   Dr AB Road, Worli, Mumbai-400018

Tel : +91-22-4974308/4944624
Fax: +91-22-4950723

2. **Organisation of Pharmaceutical Producers of India**
Cook's Building, 324,
Dr Dadabhay Naroji Road, Mumbai-400 001
Tel : +91-22-2045509, 2044518
Fax : 0+91-22-2044705

3. **Bulk Drug Manufacturers Association**
A-24, 2nd floor, View Towers,
Lakadi Ka Pul, Hyderabad-500004
Tel : 3322142 /3316328

4. **All India Small Scale Pharmaceutical Manufacturers Association**
26, Bhargav Lane, Vivil Line,
Nityanand Marg, Delhi-54
Tel : +91-11-2919140, 2918567
Fax : +91-11-2524302, 2937857

5. **Federation of Indian Chambers of Commerce and Industry**
Federation House
Tansen Marg, New Delhi-110001
Tel : +91-11-3738760-70
Fax: +91-11-3320714,3721504

6. **Confederation of Indian Industry**
23, Industrial Area
Lodi Estate, New Delhi-110 003
Tel : +91-11-4621874, 4629994-7
Fax: +91-11-4633168, 4626149

Latin Abbreviations of Some Terminologies

Abbreviation	*Meaning*	*Latin*
ad.lib.	freely as wanted	*ad libitum*
aq	water	*aqua*
bid.	twice a day	*bis in die*

Contd...

Abbreviation	*Meaning*	*Latin*
cap.	capsule	*capula*
c with bar on top	with	*cum*
div.	divide	*divide*
eq pts.	equal parts	*equalis partis*
gtt	a drop	*gutta*
h	hour	*hora*
no	number	*numero*
O	pint	*octarius*
prn	as occasion requires	*pro re nata*
qs	a sufficient quantity	*quantum sufficiat*
q4h	every 4 hours	*quaque 4 hora*
q6h	every 6 hours	*quaque 6 hora*
q1d	every day	*quaque 1 die*
q1w	every week	
qid.	four times a day	*quater in die*
sid.	once a day	*semel in die*
Sig., S.	write on the label	*signa*
stat.	immediately	*statim*
tab.	a tablet	*tabella*
tid.	three times a day	*ter in die*

Index